Insider's Guide *to*
SAVING MONEY
at the Dentist

A dentist's advice on how to effectively create and keep an amazing smile

Dr. Carson Calderwood

Transformation Media Books
Bloomington, Indiana

Published by Transformation Media Books, USA

Transformation Media Books

www.TransformationMediaBooks.com
info@TransformationMediaBooks.com

An imprint of Pen & Publish, Inc.
www.PenandPublish.com
Bloomington, Indiana
(314) 827-6567

Print ISBN: 978-1-941799-46-8
e-book ISBN: 978-1-941799-47-5

To Marisa, my peak inspiration

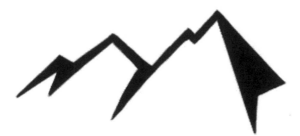

Contents

Chapter 1: Introduction 7

Chapter 2: How to Choose a Provider 11

Chapter 3: Technology in the Modern Dental Office and How
It Can Help You.. 23

Chapter 4: How to Avoid Dishonest or Overly Aggressive
Dentists 29

Chapter 5: Methods to Save Money... 41

Chapter 6: Good Home Care to Avoid Extra Dental Visits....... 49

Chapter 7: Common Dental Problems and Solutions 59

Chapter 8: Life Stages and Needed Dental Information 69

Chapter 9: Emergency Algorithm 81

Chapter 10: Common Misconceptions...................................... 85

Chapter 11: Dental Insurance.. 97

Chapter 12: Dental Odds and Ends 103

Chapter 13: Conclusion.. 113

Appendix A: Definitions 115

Appendix B: Tables.. 121

Chapter 1

Introduction

What motivated me to write this book? There are two primary reasons.

First, I deeply desire that dentistry's excellent reputation for honesty and patient care be firmly reinstated in everyone's mind. I'm very happy that so many dentists before me have done such a great job to establish dentistry as a trusted and respected profession.

Second, educating the general population to understand what their options are helps hold the dental field accountable. We live in an information age where greater transparency is expected. Access to previously hidden information because of the internet has completely changed my life for the better. My goal is to put information about quality dental work into everyone's hands to achieve even greater transparency in dentistry than already exists.

Is this information always necessary? Fortunately not very often, but there are times when people are taken advantage of. Some offices push people into treatment they don't need. Other times offices do downright dishonest work—they tell a patient he needs a crown when he needed nothing more than a simple filling. Furthermore, sometimes offices continuously put out poor work, but it doesn't show up as problematic for a couple of years. When the dental work does go bad, the patient has often forgotten which tooth was worked on or the dentist has even moved. Here are a couple examples that I have seen firsthand.

A patient came to my office with four implants placed recently in another state. Three of the implants were so far out of alignment that it would have been impossible to restore them without having the tooth stick almost straight out of his face! Furthermore, the implants were placed so close together that they couldn't have had a normal-sized crown on them. In the end, this man spent over nine thousand dollars on implants he couldn't use. He would need to spend a few more thousand dollars to have them removed and be where he was before the implants were placed!

Another patient came to me with an existing treatment plan from another office. She had heard rumors that the office she went to overtreated, so she wanted a second opinion. After doing a thorough exam, I informed her that she only needed two fillings. Frequently offices differ slightly on fillings depending on how conservative or aggressive they are, but to tell a patient that she needs two root canals and four crowns when there was absolutely no need was appalling.

I have talked to a few people who worked at an office that required their staff to make all new patients over the age of eighteen get a deep cleaning—no matter how clean their teeth were. Deep cleanings are reserved for a specific set of patients meeting strict requirements. The decision needs to be made on a case-by-case basis; currently the average dental practice has about 20% of their patients get a deep cleaning. Setting an age as the only requirement is insurance fraud and dishonest. Fortunately this is just the minority, but offices that grossly overtreat do exist. Thus, you need to know how to recognize them, even ones that only do it a little. This book will give you information to help protect your family and loved ones from offices that would take advantage of your lack of knowledge.

It is my hope that the information presented in this book will save your family thousands of dollars over the extent of your dental lives. Not only do I hope that it will help you avoid unnecessary dental treatments, but that you will be empowered to make the best choices to minimize your amount of dental work throughout your life. Once enamel has been removed, it never comes back. Therefore drilling on a tooth is always a one-way road. This book will help you travel down that road as infrequently as possible.

As you read, remember that I have some important definitions in the glossary (found in the back of this book). You will likely need to check these references frequently for definitions of several technical dental words. Check there if you come across something you don't know while reading this book or during your dental research and office visits. There are also several references to other chapters for more detailed explanations. Together, all these references will help you feel more comfortable discussing dentistry with your dental office. You will make more confident decisions as you research dentistry and develop a better idea of what you want for your oral health.

Enjoy reading and have a beautiful, truly happy smile!

Chapter 2

How to Choose a Provider

Let's start off with information on how to choose an office. Choosing the right office makes your task of choosing what dental treatments to accept much easier—you will have confidence that what you are being presented is accurate and grounded in your best interest, not the financial interest of the office. There are four criteria to find your prospective dental office: your insurance company's preferred provider list, subjective information via word of mouth (either in person or online), objective research (membership in organizations, accomplishments, office website, etc.), and a visit to the office in person.

If you want exceptional treatment whether or not it is covered by insurance, or you do not have dental insurance, then the first step doesn't matter. If insurance does matter to you, it is the best place to start because it narrows down your list of potential offices quickly and easily. Most dental insurance providers have a website to type in your zip code, including a mileage radius that you are willing to travel. This online tool will immediately create a list of all dental offices within those search parameters. Like I said above, it is quick and easy! But, this doesn't have to be a limiting factor in your search. For more detailed information on dental offices, insurance companies, and exploring your options, see Chapter 11: Dental Insurance.

The next step is to search for subjective information about the potential offices. People usually recommend dentists based on how the dentist or hygienist makes them feel, not necessarily on the quality of work. Therefore, if an office consistently treats people poorly you will receive that feedback. However, it can be harder to tell if a dentist does quality work. Luckily, the process to become a dentist is strenuous enough that there are not many that fall into that category. They do exist, but it is easy to steer clear of them with a little online research. The question then becomes whether this dentist will consistently meet your demands for what you want in a dental provider, not just occasionally or most of the time. An easy way to make sure they are consistently doing acceptable work is to check online reviews.

Online reviews are helpful, and it is definitely the best place to start your search, but they must be taken with a grain of salt. It is easy to type the doctor's name into a search engine and read the available information. This is why it is a great place to start in your hunt for a dental office. At the same time, it is easy for an office to ask friends and family to write positive reviews. Because these reviews obviously aren't going to be negative, I recommend steering clear of an office that has a significant amount of negative reviews.

That being said, don't ignore an office if it has one or two negative reviews, especially if there are several positive ones. Consider the ratio of negative to positive reviews, and pay particular attention to the comments in the negative reviews. It is impossible to make everyone happy. Every business will have someone who didn't like how things were done, no matter how great their customer service is. Keep in mind that if there are only three reviews and one is bad, that it is likely an indicator that people aren't feeling strongly enough about the office doing exceptional work to go online and share their opinion with the world. The office might not be terrible, but they probably aren't exceptional—and you deserve exceptional. I recommend that you only patronize businesses that do exceptional work. Don't settle on mediocre work when exceptional is available. Hopefully, the mediocre offices will be encouraged to change when they lose patronage.

In addition to online research, ask your friends and neighbors. This usually isn't as effective as your online search because most people will not have thoroughly researched as you did. They probably just went to the most visible dentist due to either location or advertising. As long as they don't have a negative experience, they continue to go there and claim to have a great dentist. Like I stated earlier, most people judge their dentist on how nice they are and not on whether the quality of work is good.

Now is a good time to talk about how to judge the quality of work done by a dentist. It can be very hard to tell if a dentist's work is high quality. The best way would be to follow all treatment done over a ten-year period and compare the rate of failed restorations to industry standards. For example, for veneers, the industry standard is a 93% success rate at ten years.[1] You obviously don't have ten years to wait and see how your local dentist is doing. That also means seven out of every one hundred will have failed for a competent dentist. In other words, for every two patients that get six veneers (common set of teeth visible in a person's smile), at least one will fail prematurely. Typically, that means that one will break or fall off before twenty years, the normal lifespan of a dental restoration.

This brings us to two important points. First, even good work done by the best dentist will have some failures. These failures may be due to a myriad of causes, anywhere from the patient's fault to the doctor's fault, or there are unknown causes that are not the fault of anyone. The key is to find a dentist who understands the potential failures and does what is necessary to avoid as many as possible. Secondly, it is important to know there are certain expectations of excellence that should be achieved. Twenty years ago, a success rate of 93% for veneers would have seemed impossible to some. With today's technology and expe-

---

1 Layton, D., Walton, T. (2007). An up to 16-year prospective study of 304 porcelain veneers. *Int J Prosthodont*, 20.4, 389–96. http://www.ncbi.nlm.nih.gov/pubmed/17695870.

rience, you can achieve much better results than were possible even ten years ago!

So, what can you do? As stated earlier, you can usually avoid those that do terrible work by checking online reviews. It is easy to tell when someone does a poor job, especially if they consistently do poor work. It is a little harder to tell the difference between good and great. One approach is to call the local or state Dental Society and ask if they have any complaints about the doctor in question. You can also search the state's quality control board website to see if the dentist has any license restrictions or past lawsuits for malpractice.

The third step in our research process is also an indirect way to predict if a dentist's work will be good or great. Look at the office's website or even call and ask to find out what type of post-graduate education the doctor has taken. Dental schools typically only teach basic and fundamental treatment skills. Dental school is four years long and does not provide enough time to get a deep understanding of advanced techniques or modern dentistry methods and materials. Some schools will give a small amount of training, but definitely not an in-depth experience. Fortunately, state dental boards require a certain amount of yearly continuing education hours to ensure dentists are keeping up with changes that occur. For example, the state of Washington, where I practice, requires that I get twenty-one credit hours every year. It can be hard to close the office and pay to take those courses instead of working, but it is always worth the effort. If doctors dedicate themselves to a decent amount of learning, especially in the first few years out of school, they will often get double or triple the minimum requirement of continuing education hours each year.

Now you may ask if it is acceptable to see a dentist who is fresh out of school. There is a huge variance from one dentist to another at graduation time. After about three to five years that difference shrinks. On-the-job training comes at you pretty fast and hard when you graduate. Most new graduates will do a fine job of routine treatments, such as finding cavities and filling them. Experience and extra education really come into play with things like advanced crown and bridge work or TMJ problems. Those treatments can be very complicated and definitely require extra training to do them well. If you go to a practice that has more than one doctor, and the younger doctor works on your teeth, I wouldn't worry for routine treatment and exams. If you have more complicated treatments, it would be a good choice to see the more experienced doctor.

The final step of your research process is visiting the dental office and asking about their education or other questions you may have. Your list of offices to interview shouldn't be too large; you may even skip this step if you feel like you have enough information on your prospective dentist. If your list is still too long, consider widening your word-of-mouth sources for opinions about those offices on your list. Other people to ask would include your physician, pediatrician, or local pharmacist. If you still are looking to narrow your list, think of "must-have" criteria you would like in your dental office. Examples include office hours, days open, handicap accessibility, or whether children are seen.

Call the office(s) you would like to visit and ask for either an office tour or a chance to meet and talk with the dentist. If the office is not accommodating, then this could be a red flag that keeps you from wanting to visit them anyway. Your office visit doesn't have to be formal; it may just involve a quick look to see the office and meet the dentist and staff. Often the front office staff are more than willing to take time to answer your questions. Here are some example questions to ask or thoughts to consider when visiting an office:

- How do they handle after-hour emergency visits?
- What payment options do they have?
- Does the office seem clean and well sterilized?
- If you have children that you plan on taking to this office, how friendly are the office and staff toward children?
- What is the policy on missed appointments?
- Does the technology seem to be up to date?

Overall, there are three main areas a dentist should excel in when you are making the decision of which office to choose:

1. Having your best interest in mind and not focusing on sales or pushing unnecessary treatments.
2. Doing work at a high level of workmanship and in a nice, professional manner.
3. Having an office that is kept clean and sterile.

Meeting those three most important criteria ensures that you will get high quality work done in a pleasing way without unnecessary treatment. You get only what you need, you get it done well, and you enjoy the experience as much as possible.

You see more than just the dentist when you go to the dental office. In my office, I try very hard to make sure I have very proficient and friendly hygienists and front office staff. They are the people that you will interact with most. They are the true face of my practice. Not only should you evaluate a potential practice based on the dentist, but you should also evaluate the other staff. In some instances, when specialty work is needed, you will also need to evaluate a specialist. The remaining part of this chapter will discuss how to evaluate specialists and determine what each person's job is.

Hygiene

A hygienist is the person who will usually do your cleanings. Hygienists typically complete two extra years of training beyond a bachelor's degree. The main body of their studies is concerned with general and advanced cleanings, with most programs offering some training in giving anesthetic injections and placing fillings. In some states the hygienist can do extra procedures, such as placing a filling. They can't drill out a cavity, but after the dentist has done that, they can place the restoration. Not very many offices take advantage of this; patients find it unusual since they traditionally expect the dentist to do it. If the restoration is placed by a hygienist, no matter how well it is done, patients will wonder if it was done properly. To avoid this potential fear and frustration, most offices skip utilizing the hygienist. Often a hygienist will be used to administer a local anesthesia, especially when the doctor is running behind.

Choosing a hygienist mostly comes down to your personal cleaning-style preference and personality, unless you need advanced cleanings. Most hygienists get more than enough training to take care of their patients. Since you typically spend more time with them than anyone else in a dental office, it is nice to be treated by someone whom you enjoy being with. Another cleaning-style preference to consider is the speed of the hygienist. Some hygienists work fast, some work slowly. You may prefer one type of cleaning to the other.

Beyond that, hygienists typically fall into one of two categories, heavy-handed or light. Heavy-handed hygienists make sure to get every last bit of tartar off your teeth. Sometimes that can be more painful. I personally feel that getting the last 2% of a 100% perfectly clean mouth causes 75% of the pain resulting from a cleaning. For that reason, I personally prefer light-handed hygienists, especially considering that I don't have any periodontal problems and I come in regularly for cleanings. That may leave my teeth only 98% clean, but it also leaves me with 75% less pain! On the other hand, I have some patients that feel if the cleaning didn't hurt then their teeth weren't properly cleaned. Understand which type of cleaning you prefer and ask how the office's hygienist typically works. This is especially true if the office has more than one hygienist. Find out which one works more in line with what you prefer and request to see that one.

Dental Specialists

There are six types of dental specialists that you are likely to see. I will cover what each one specializes in later, but specialists are dentists who have completed extra schooling to perform an advanced level of dental treatment in that area. Specialists also can have some specialized equipment that might not be cost effective for a general dentist to purchase since they are not doing as many of those procedures as the specialist does. For the most part, a general dentist can do any treatment that a specialist does. For example, many dentists do root canals, but often they will send complex cases to an endodontist. This ensures that you get the treatment done well and quickly. Even if the general dentist could do the treatment, it often takes them significantly longer to complete. They give you the referral to save you time and to ensure that you get the treatment done correctly. Because there are so many different areas of treatment in dentistry, from dentures to implants or from root canals to cosmetics, it is fairly unlikely to excel in every area. Most general dentists choose different aspects of dentistry that they enjoy; they learn to do those procedures well and send you off to a specialist for those they don't know as well.

You deserve a word of warning here. As we have mentioned previously, not every dentist has your best interest at heart. Some offices might avoid sending you to a specialist when they should. They do that for one reason—to keep the work and money in their office. As I go through the various treatments each specialty focuses on, you will be able to better predict which procedures will likely need to be referred elsewhere. If you need one of those procedures done, ask your dentist what kind of warranty they offer, what complications could possibly arise, and how they would deal with those complications. That being said, there are also complications that can arise which are out of the dentist's control. Knowing whether a specialist should do a procedure can be hard to figure out. Having a dentist you trust in the first place is the best way to avoid this problem.

Usually, when it comes time to get treatment from a dental specialist you will receive a referral from your general dentist or hygienist. Again, having an office you trust makes this decision easy because you know they are sending you somewhere to receive the best care. You don't have to fear that the dentist has an incentive to send you anywhere. Not only is it unethical, it is also illegal to receive kickbacks. Thankfully, I've never heard of this actually happening.

Most specialists do great work anyway, especially when it comes to routine treatments. To get into a specialty school you have to perform in the top percent of your dental class. Being accepted into a specialty school proves the dentist is one of the best. Then, the dentist receives a few years of specialty training in an area of expertise. They become like a very finely tuned instrument. For common treatments, most people choose a dental specialist based on location and insurance coverage.

For the more complex treatments or unusual treatments it still can be good to evaluate your options and get different opinions before deciding on what treatment to do. For example, if you need a tooth pulled or a root canal, then going to any oral surgeon or endodontist respectively, will be fine. On the other hand, if you need mandibular advancement surgery or post-traumatic replacement of the maxillary anterior arch with implants, then choosing the right person within a specialty can be paramount.

The following table shows the six most common specialists and what they do in layman's terms.

Specialty	Description
Oral surgeon	Also known as an oral maxillofacial surgeon (OMS). They specialize in surgical procedures on the head and neck area. There is a significant amount of overlap between an OMS and an Ear, Nose, and Throat physician. People primarily go to oral surgeons for wisdom teeth extractions. Similarly, people go for complex extractions of other teeth and evaluations for abnormal growths or diseases in the head and neck area.

Endodontist	Endodontists specialize in doing root canals very well. If you have tooth pain that can't be figured out, then your dentist may send you here to rule out the need for a root canal.
Orthodontist	Orthodontists straighten teeth with braces. Because they primarily work with teenagers, they also are highly trained in growth and development.
Pedodontist	Pedodontists specialize in the treatment of children. Children do not have to be seen by a pedodontist, but some families choose to send their children to a pedodontist until they turn eighteen, at which point they transition to a general practice.
Periodontist	Periodontists focus on the periodontum. The periodontum is the soft and hard tissue of the mouth, in other words, the gums and bones. They mainly see patients for two things: 1) treating people with periodontal disease and 2) performing surgeries on the gums or bone. There is some overlap with oral surgeons.
Prosthodontist	A prosthodontist has advanced education in mainly crown, bridge, and denture treatments. If you need several crowns or a very complex bridge, then your dentist might refer you to a prosthodontist.

As you can see, choosing a dentist that you trust goes a long way to ensuring that you get high quality and only necessary work done, whether it is in their office or a specialist's office. Put your time in at the beginning to find a good dentist, and then you can trust that you aren't paying for unnecessary treatment or getting an unacceptable quality of work done.

Chapter 3

Technology in the Modern Dental Office and How It Can Help You

Technology in dentistry is changing quickly and drastically. Everything in our world is becoming digital. Once something is digitized, the information can quickly and easily be shared, stored, altered, etc. It really is a wonderful thing in many instances. For example, your average digital intraoral x-ray uses about 90% less radiation than the film ones used on me as a child in the 1980s. (See Chapter 10: Common Misconceptions, for more information on x-rays.) In this chapter I will go through some common technologies in dentistry and discuss how they help you get better, quicker, and easier treatment. You can use this information to help decide which offices to visit and which treatments to get done.

Lasers

There are three lasers commonly used in dental offices. Starting with the smallest, the DIAGNOdent laser is used for cavity detection. Many offices utilize this technology to help change cavity detection from a subjective process done by the dentist to an objective process that doesn't vary. They can run this little laser over the teeth and get density readings of specific teeth. Readings above a certain number (higher numbers equal lower density) are very often a sure bet that you have a cavity.

This is helpful because you can get a cavity that starts deep in the very bottom of a fissure (groove) and doesn't grow sideways to become visible. Once a cavity penetrates through enamel into the dentin, it can grow faster and enlarge before being visible in the mouth or on x-rays. This laser cavity detection provides a visual down into the bottom of those very tiny fissures and detects decay that would otherwise be impossible to find. The result is that the dentist can catch the cavity earlier to avoid a root canal or crown, thus saving you a significant amount of money and tooth structure.

The second laser commonly used in a dental office is a soft tissue laser. These lasers are more powerful than the ones used to find cavities and can cut or "melt" soft tissues. They are used instead of scalpels for surgeries where it is necessary to trim back gums. Soft tissue lasers can be better than using a scalpel because it cauterizes the tissue as it cuts, and therefore stops all the bleeding that a traditional scalpel would create. There are several other treatments that can be done with this type of laser, such as decreasing healing time of canker sores (aphthous ulcers) or periodontal disease.

One nice benefit of the above two lasers is that they are not very expensive. Thus, many dental offices are able to incorporate them into their practices. The third type of commonly used laser is much more expensive: a hard tissue laser. These lasers can cut soft tissue like the soft tissue laser, but they are also powerful enough to cut through natural tooth structure. One of the benefits to these lasers is that cavities can often be removed without anesthesia! Besides the downside of the cost, there are two other negatives. Because these lasers can't cut through metal, you have to take away more good tooth structure than you would have had you removed a silver filling with a traditional drill. This less conservative approach can be a deal breaker for many offices. Also, the laser doesn't always require that the tooth be numb, but too often it does, which is discouraging if you were expecting to skip the needle. These negatives keep many offices from using this type of laser for fillings. Some offices will use them for periodontal work, usually periodontists.

In-Office Porcelain Work

There are now several companies selling equipment that allows dentists to provide same-day porcelain restorations, such as crowns. The big upside to this technology is that you can get a crown done in one visit and skip getting numb twice or wearing a temporary crown. You don't have to return for a second visit. The dentist takes "digital impressions" of your teeth by taking 3D images with a camera. The computer then takes this information and with the skill of the dentist and his staff, a new crown can be made on the computer to fit your tooth perfectly. This information is sent to a CAD/CAM machine that uses diamond cutters to cut your crown out of a block of porcelain. There are various sizes and colors of blocks that can be used.

This also works for veneers, onlays, and inlays. For the most part, the porcelain restorations are equal in quality but not quite as good looking as those made by hand in a dental lab. For that reason this technology is most commonly used only on posterior teeth. Front teeth that are visible when you smile will therefore still be sent to a lab to fabricate your crown or veneer. That could all change soon as this technology is improving every year. Companies are starting to integrate the data from 3D x-rays with this machine to make fairly fool-proof implant placement systems. Digitizing your x-rays and photos will provide more improvements in quality and shorten the visit time when it comes to dental work in the future.

X-rays

Digital x-rays have changed the dental field in much the same way that digital cameras have changed photography. Instead of taking an image and waiting to see whether you got what you wanted, you can know instantly. Then if you did get the x-ray you wanted, you can save it forever on a backup system or email it to anyone, anywhere in the world! It can be enlarged on a monitor to see what the dentist is seeing. Also, the dentist can change the contrast or colorize the black and white image to allow you to see the cavity. Being part of the diagnosis process in this way can help you feel confident in the dentist's prognosis of a cavity, rather than watching your dentist look at a little film and tell you there is a cavity that you can't even see.

Because digital x-ray sensors can be more sensitive than film, a much smaller dosage of radiation is required. This greatly reduces your level of exposure to the equivalent amount that you would get from spending a few hours in the sun or taking a plane ride. I will discuss more about radiation exposure in Chapter 10: Common Misconceptions.

Three-dimensional x-rays are on the horizon of becoming standard in all dental offices. That is where the computer takes all of the data from the sensor and can manipulate that into a three-dimensional rendering of the scanned area. This can greatly help in diagnosing. For example, someone may have a small crack on a root that perpetually causes pain. Getting a root canal won't fix the problem. Looking at a standard two-dimensional x-ray won't show anything in most cases. This uncommon problem can continue for years causing constant pain. Using a 3D x-ray system can allow for better viewing of individual roots and the ability to diagnose a root fracture, thus avoiding costly treatments that won't actually help.

Digital Charts

Digital charting has more of an indirect benefit to you as a dental patient. First, it shows that your office is staying current and not stuck in dentistry of twenty or more years ago. Digital charts make sharing and storing your information much easier. You should be able to request free copies to keep for yourself, if you want. If you move, it only takes a minute to send all the x-rays and chart notes to the new office. If you need a root canal, they can email your x-rays and information to the specialist so they don't have to take as many x-rays, reducing your costs and radiation exposure. If the office happens to have the unfortunate experience of burning down or flooding, off-site backups of the database can be easily restored, and no information is lost.

In summary, dentistry is moving with the world into the digital age. Once digitized, the data can be easily evaluated, shared, stored, manipulated, etc. Also, with technological advancements in lasers, treatment can be done with shorter healing times and less anesthesia.

Chapter 4

How to Avoid Dishonest or Overly Aggressive Dentists

This chapter, probably more than any other, will help you avoid paying for dentistry that you don't need. An important point to clarify first is that there is a spectrum of aggressive dentists. On the far left there are dentists trying to be ultra conservative; they don't do treatments that should be done. For instance, if a dentist waits too long to fix a cavity, a root canal will be necessary. Fixing the small cavity would cost about 20% of the price of a root canal, and often with a root canal, you also need a buildup and a crown. In that case, the small filling would have only been 10% of what you end up spending for the root canal, buildup, and crown. Being too conservative can cost you a lot of money.

On the other end of the spectrum there are dentists who do treatment that isn't needed. Dentists do this either because they are choosing to dishonestly make more money or they have a treatment philosophy of overdoing things for what they view as better results. It can be difficult to determine the dentist's motive unless there is gross overtreatment being done.

So where is the happy medium? That really depends on your philosophy as a patient. I often compare the mouth to a car. Do you have a nice car that you wash frequently, change the oil every three thousand miles, and repair at the dealership with new factory parts? On the other hand, do you have an old car, go several thousand miles before changing the oil, and always repair it on your own or at the cheapest repair place with parts from a wrecking yard? Those are two very different cars, but they both get you to work. Also, it can be good to compare your mouth to your overall health. Do you make organic green smoothies for breakfast every morning and stay out of the sun to reduce your risk of skin cancer or do you smoke frequently and eat at least one meal a day at a fast-food restaurant? Are you a nice-car-and-smoothies-for-breakfast person or a used-car-and-eat-whatever-you-desire person?

If these two different people had a silver filling that started to show visible fracture lines, they would react very differently. The first example is a person whose happy medium is more along the lines of removing the amalgam and placing a porcelain restoration to avoid any fracture of the tooth. In reality, they probably would have replaced the amalgam with white porcelain long before the expanding amalgam had enough time to create the fracture lines. The second person is likely to wait until the tooth breaks before replacing the old amalgam. Since the risk of the tooth breaking completely and needing extraction is small, they will wait for the tooth to need repair. Both are acceptable philosophies. One is much more preventative than the other. Finding a dentist who matches your dental philosophy and will treat you according to your dental philosophy will help you avoid dentists who treat more aggressively or conservatively than you want.

Examples

So, what are some pitfalls that people can fall into when they end up paying for unnecessary dental treatments? You will rarely be told to avoid treatment that you absolutely need. The pitfalls usually come from getting more treatment done than needed. The following list explains the most common overtreatments, when treatment is necessary, and how you could be enticed into getting work done when it isn't needed.

Being told you need a deep cleaning:

What is it?

A deep cleaning is also known as scaling and root planing (or SRP). This cleaning is more involved and complex than a regular cleaning. It often can take more than one visit and require anesthesia due to the pain it can cause while being performed.

When is it necessary?

This procedure is necessary when you have gone a long time without a cleaning and there is a significant amount of tartar (calculus) built up. There are also people who are more prone to buildup and need more frequent and deeper cleanings than the average person. This is especially necessary when you have had some bone loss due to a significant amount of calculus. Because more work is involved, the American Dental Association (ADA) has created a billing code to differentiate the amount of work required for a deeper cleaning from the amount of work required for a regular cleaning. Most insurance companies don't cover deep cleanings at 100% like they do for regular cleanings. However, once you have completed the deep cleaning, they will usually cover the more expensive periodontal maintenance cleanings at 100% and allow one or two extra cleanings a year. Therefore they typically happen every four or six months, but in severe cases, cleanings can happen every three months.

How could you be tricked into getting it?

Everybody experiences a buildup of calculus on teeth. Most people don't floss regularly and can have 4–5 mm periodontal pockets around some of their teeth. Just having those two conditions doesn't always mean a deep cleaning is necessary. If you have so much calculus and stain that the scraping (and/or ultrasonic cleaning) part of your cleaning takes longer than thirty to forty minutes, then you are in need of a deep cleaning. You would also need a deep cleaning if you have a significant amount of bone loss or gum problems. If you have numerous 5 mm or deeper pockets, for example, you would require an advanced cleaning. Basically, if you are told you need a deep cleaning, ask why a regular cleaning won't suffice. Overly aggressive offices will tell you that you need a deep cleaning because not only does insurance pay more for the procedure, but it also allows all your follow-up cleanings to be periodontal maintenance instead of a regular prophy (name for regular cleaning). Periodontal maintenance has a higher charge and is usually 100% covered. So, if an office can get you to pay a little extra for that first cleaning, they can continue to get more money from every cleaning. Even though those following cleanings are 100% covered, this scenario can become a negative to you if you need extra work done. For example, if you need two crowns, but you have already used up your insurance with the more costly periodontal maintenance cleanings.

Being told you need to replace a filling, especially an amalgam (silver) filling:

What is it?

For various reasons you may be advised to replace your old or silver fillings with white ones. Some reasons are legitimate, some are not, and some are dependent on your preferences. As with everything, you should know the pros and cons to getting the procedure done so that you can decide if it is something that you should do.

When is it necessary?

Without having a cavity (tooth decay) or fracture, replacing a filling is rarely necessary. Sometimes an office will say that a filling is failing or starting to fail. You should ask for clarification if there is an actual cavity or not. Can they see the cavity on an x-ray or can they get a clinical stick when they poke into the decay with their dental instrument? If not, you might not have a legitimate cavity that needs a filling. If there is a stick, you should be able to feel the metal instrument stick into your tooth. Other times you may be told to replace a silver filling because it is leaking mercury into your body. For more on this see Chapter 10: Common Misconceptions. In short, silver fillings are not a significant source of mercury. Their biggest negative is that they expand more than your tooth does when hot. The expansion causes fracturing to occur, which eventually leads to the tooth breaking to one level or another. The second biggest negative can be aesthetics.

How could you be tricked into getting it?

Offices will play up the mercury myth to make you feel a strong desire to replace them with white fillings. They may also tell you that fracture lines mean you have to replace the filling. As described in the beginning of this chapter, that depends more on your preferences than actual needs. If the tooth hurts or is broken, then replacing the filling because of fracture lines is a good idea. A bad-looking filling may or may not mean it should be replaced. Is it a white filling that has just turned yellow or has a little bit of stain on its edge where it meets the tooth? Those usually don't require replacement. Is there a lot of darkness under a white filling that used to not be there or is an old white filling crumbling? Those would require replacement. It can be hard to tell when you should and when you shouldn't and may come down to preventative preferences. Be wary that your dentist is overtreating and having you do unnecessary dental work if you are frequently being told one of the reasons listed above.

Being told you need a filling because there is a dark spot on an x-ray or a dark spot visually on a tooth:

What is it?

Cavities show up on x-rays usually as dark triangles with the base of the triangle being on the outside of the tooth pointing in. Cavities show up clinically (visually in the mouth) usually as dark areas that are soft and sticky when poked into with a dental instrument called an explorer.

When is it necessary?

A common rule of thumb for cavities found on x-rays is that if the tip of that triangle is more than halfway to the dentin (tooth structure under the enamel) then a filling should be placed. Often you can have a little bit of darkness show up from the start of a cavity that could stop (arrested decay) or it could be an old arrested cavity. These cavities are created from not flossing enough. If you start to clean well before the cavity gets too big, then it can soak up calcium and fluoride from your saliva and re-solidify or stop progressing. (See Chapter 10: Common Misconceptions for what a cavity actually is and a more detailed explanation of fluoride.) Similarly, you may see a dark spot in one of your teeth. That could be a cavity, arrested decay, or just a stain. If it isn't soft or sticky when poked, then you don't need a filling. As always, if it bothers you aesthetically, then definitely get the filling, but don't feel pressure to get it replaced otherwise.

How could you be tricked into getting it?

You can be told that any dark spot is a cavity because teeth are supposed to be white. Ask for clarification if something is just stain or potentially arrested decay. If they can explain to you that it is more, then feel justified in getting the work done. This usually will manifest when someone suddenly needs lots of fillings that weren't previously there or when a dentist diagnoses more fillings than you used to get at another dentist. (However, it is possible the previous dentist wasn't diagnosing decay like they should have.)

Being told you need a crown or onlay instead of a filling:

What is it?

A crown will cover most to all of a tooth with strong porcelain or metal such as gold. An onlay will be smaller and cover less of the tooth, but it will replace at least one cusp.

When is it necessary?

Crowns and onlays are usually necessary when the filling gets too big and the material isn't able to support the forces applied to the tooth. This usually happens when the filling covers more than half of the tooth. Sometimes an onlay is needed even if less than half the tooth is being replaced, or if you have large fracture lines caused by a small silver filling.

How could you be tricked into getting it?

If you don't meet the restoration size description in the previous paragraph, but you are told a crown or onlay is necessary. It is possible to need a crown or onlay even if you don't have a tooth with a filling. If you have Cracked Tooth Syndrome or get a root canal, a crown is very necessary. Ask your doctor if it is possible to just get a filling. In the case of onlays, a composite filling can often work though not as well. Again, deciding which to get may come down to what type of dentistry you prefer.

Being told you need a build-up with your crown:

What is it?

A build-up is a restoration needed on top of a tooth that doesn't have enough structure to hold a crown without it falling off. The build-up is usually made of a composite or similar material that will chemically bond to the tooth.

When is it necessary?

If your tooth has a large cavity or especially if it had a root canal and breaks off flat at the gum line. If you do get a crown, it likely will come off very soon because there isn't much tooth structure for the crown to adhere to. To avoid that problem the dentist will place a filling on the tooth that microscopically locks into the tooth. Then the crown can be glued onto that build-up to give a better overall restoration.

How could you be tricked into getting it?

Some offices will by default say every crown needs a build-up, even when they aren't needed. If you are being charged to get build-up in addition to your crown and you don't think you are missing a large portion of your tooth, ask the dentist if the crown could be placed without doing the build-up. You need a minimal amount of tooth sticking out of the gums to have a crown stay on. You usually need 1.5 mm or more of space for the new crown between your tooth and the tooth it hits when your mouth is closed. The requirements make it difficult to decide if you really do need a build-up. Just ask your dentist to explain why yours is needed.

Being told you need a root canal when you don't:

What is it?

A root canal is a procedure where the dentist uses files to clean out the canals on a tooth and refills the hole with a filling.

When is it necessary?

A root canal is necessary when you have a cavity or broken tooth that goes all the way to the nerve canal. There is at least one canal or hole in every tooth. Every canal has a blood vessel and a nerve inside it. The nerve then sends small nerve endings out into the dentin of the tooth. If bacteria get into the canal, they easily travel down and infect the bone. The body cannot get rid of the infection due to the low amount of blood flow in the blood vessel of the canal. Therefore, you have to file the walls of the canal to remove the bacteria in it, disinfect, and refill with a rubber-like material.

How could you be tricked into getting it?

There are two main overtreatments that occur. First, sometimes it can be difficult to tell if a root canal is necessary. Overly aggressive doctors will just suggest doing a root canal in questionable times instead of waiting or doing other tests. There have been times when people have gotten a root canal when all they had was a sinus infection (these two instances can mimic each other). The best, although not foolproof, test that your dentist should do is a cold test. They should put something very cold on the tooth and count how long you feel the cold or pain. The following responses give their respective diagnosis:

- 0–5 seconds = Normal tooth
- 5–10 seconds = Irritation that will likely go away if the problem is fixed (i.e., do a filling or take anti-inflammatory pills)
- 10+ seconds = Past the point of no return, needs root canal
- No response = Likely a dead tooth or poorly done test. If the test was done well and there was no response, then the nerve is completely dead in the tooth from a long-standing infection and a root canal should be done.

The second situation where root canals are often overtreated occurs when you are getting a filling done. When drilling out a cavity, if the cavity is too big the dentist will drill all the way to that canal and hit the blood vessel. This is called an exposure. For many years the standard was to get a root canal if this occurs. Modern dentistry with a focus on conservative treatment has done research on whether small pinpoint exposures really require a root canal. Fortunately, these studies show that in many cases the tooth will be fine if a medicine is placed over the exposure and then a filling placed. This is because the tooth can actually repair itself on the inside! The size of the exposure and how long the bacteria exposure lasted can vary, so it doesn't always turn out fine. Other research has shown that if you laser that exposure with a soft tissue laser, as well as place the medicine and a filling, your chances diminish even more for needing a root canal. This process will kill any bacteria in the area and sterilize the exposure. The aforementioned example is yet another reason to make sure you are visiting a dentist with an understanding of modern dentistry and the equipment.

Being told you need a crown on an anterior tooth that received a root canal:

When is it necessary?

Often when you get a root canal you should get a crown. This is very true on back teeth that receive very strong forces during chewing or clenching. I have seen a few teeth break right in half just after a person received a root canal because they chose not to get the crown. It is always sad because they recently spent good money on a root canal and now they have to pay more money to get the tooth extracted.

How could you be tricked into getting it?

Basically understanding when it is necessary and when it isn't will help you know if you are being pushed into too aggressive dentistry. Anterior teeth, from canine to canine, that have a very small hole drilled into them are usually fine without a crown. If you had a large break, cavity, or large root canal, then you likely will need a crown. First premolars are in the middle when it comes to needing crowns after root canals and anything posterior to that should often get a crown.

Dishonest dental work can happen in so many ways it would be hard for me to list them all and explain how to tell the difference between actually needing it or not. This chapter has listed the most common ones. While writing this book I heard a disheartening story from a hygienist about a dishonest dentist she had previously worked for. The hygienist had taken an x-ray, and it was clearly visible that the tooth had an abscess. In that situation there is only two options. You either do a root canal or extract the tooth. In this case the dentist recommended the patient get a filling done first because the tooth would need a crown after the root canal was done. Insurance companies will cover a crown even if a filling was recently done. This dentist knew that she could get the extra treatment covered even though there was absolutely no need for it.

As you can see throughout this chapter sometimes recommended treatment is a matter of preference, yet sometimes you are getting treatment done that you just didn't need. Understanding what your treatment options are and why you need the treatment will help you feel more comfortable in saying yes to the dental work you need and no to the work you don't. It deserves repeating here again: the best way to ensure that you don't do unnecessary dental work is to do your homework and pick an honest dentist in the first place.

Chapter 5
Methods to Save Money

This chapter, along with Chapter 4: How to Avoid Dishonest or Overly Aggressive Dentists, and Chapter 6: Good Home Care to Avoid Extra Dental Visits, are the three chapters in this book that will help you save money when it comes to avoiding unnecessary dental work. Here we will cover the most common areas where people pay for work that they don't need at all, can forgo if they want to wait until they have more money or better insurance, or finally, avoid because they only want to do things that are absolutely necessary. With each area I will help you understand the inherent risks (if any).

The most important and easiest way to save money stems from the old adage, "An ounce of prevention is worth a pound of cure." This is definitely true in relation to saving money on dental treatments if you have insurance. That is because in most instances your insurance will cover your cleanings 100%. Getting regular cleanings will help your dentist and hygienist catch problems when they are small. Catching a cavity in between your teeth with x-rays when it is small will cost you a lot less money than not finding it until it hurts so bad that you have to get a root canal and a crown. If you don't have insurance and are paying for exams and x-rays out of pocket, you can take x-rays a little less frequently. Just remember that you are gambling a little. If you get cavities easily, then I wouldn't allow much time to pass before getting your next x-ray. You'll likely come out ahead financially by catching those cavities early, even if you are paying for a cleaning, an exam, and x-rays out of pocket. One important thing to remember is you are allowing the cavity to get bigger when you wait, even if you don't end up needing a root canal. Once enamel is removed, you never get it back. Losing as little as possible is always the better option.

If you are getting your treatment options thoroughly explained to you on larger fillings, then you will be given a choice between composite and porcelain. Both have pros and cons. Both are aesthetically pleasing in that they come in various shades of white and when done well, they can look very good. The number one benefit of a composite filling compared to porcelain is that it is cheaper. Composite fillings have two main drawbacks. Primarily, it is not as strong as porcelain. If you do very large fillings with composite, they tend to fracture easily and wear down faster. In fact, porcelain doesn't wear down since it is stronger than your teeth and could possibly wear your opposing teeth down if not polished well. Another drawback of composite is that it expands more than the tooth does when heated. The benefit to it over amalgam is that composite bonds to the tooth to help hold it together, whereas amalgam fillings just push the sides of the tooth apart and thus lead to more fractures.

In summary, very large fillings and teeth that require crowns should always get a porcelain filling. If you are interested in saving money and not getting as high quality of work done, then you can get a large composite filling instead of porcelain. But please understand you may have to replace it sooner because of early fractures. This is similar to the question of which car do you want to buy, the Honda or the Acura? Both are from the same base company, but one gets you better features for a higher price.

Prevention

A previously mentioned point I would like to stress again as a way to save money is the importance of good home care. This is by far the best way to save money on dentistry. If you brush well twice a day, floss once a day, and don't keep simple sugars on your teeth for extended periods of time, then most people will have little to no dental problems. Because it is such an important part of avoiding unnecessary dental treatments, I have dedicated an entire chapter to that discussion. (See Chapter 6: Good Home Care to Avoid Extra Dental Visits.)

Fluoride usage is another great preventative tool, and it is even a reparative tool because fluoride can help reverse minor damage. For a very detailed explanation of fluoride, see Chapter 10: Common Misconceptions. Studies have shown that small decalcifications (beginnings of a cavity) can be reversed with topical fluoride and good home care. For this reason in my office we recommend fluoride treatments when there are questionable results on x-rays or small cavities in chewing surfaces. Fluoride is cheaper than a filling and if it remineralizes the tooth then no filling is needed! You save money and enamel, which is the holy grail of dental treatment.

Sealants are also a good way to save money, especially if placed correctly on children. Children often don't have great teeth-cleaning habits; any help they get can make a big difference. A sealant fills in the natural grooves in a tooth that are hard to clean and easily harbor bacteria that cause cavities. Often the bottom of these grooves can be very thin and deep. Too deep in fact for your toothbrush bristles to properly clean. Therefore, small bits of food will stay at the bottom of those grooves and over time a cavity will develop. To avoid cavities, the dentist or one of the staff in the dental office will clean the tooth and place a sealant.

A sealant starts out as a liquid filling. It is a liquid substance so that it can easily flow down into the bottom of those grooves. Then a curing light is shined on it and the liquid filling turns hard in a few seconds. As long as it doesn't come out you can brush normally and not worry about getting a cavity in an area you previously couldn't keep clean. That is what makes the small charge for a sealant worth it. It prevents you from getting fillings that usually cost four times as much. Again, it also prevents you from having tooth structure removed that you can't get back.

Sealants can be preventative for a tooth without any existing problems, but what do you do when you get a dark spot on a tooth? Darkness can range from slight stain that comes off with a cleaning to permanent stain. Basically, if an area on your tooth is not cleaned adequately, then food particles are allowed to sit on the tooth. At first the chemicals in food that give it color (either natural or synthetic) will stain a tooth. When food particles are allowed to sit against the tooth long enough that means bacteria are able to sit there as well. As bacteria eat the sugars in your food they produce the byproduct of acid. That acid will dissolve into the tooth where the bacteria are hanging out. As they dissolve into the tooth they start to work their way inside that soft tooth structure. Food chemicals can soak into the soft structure as well, and the cavity spreads. If this process continues long enough, the bacteria will work a couple millimeters into the tooth and be out of the range of your toothbrush no matter how well you clean. At this point, the only way to fix a cavity is to drill into that soft area, remove it, and replace the hole with a filling.

Should you jump in and get a filling whenever you have stain? I personally do not think so, unless it is in an area that bothers you aesthetically. Stain can sit in the bottom of a groove, for example, on a tooth's chewing surface for decades without becoming a cavity if it is kept clean. If it is a very deep groove that your toothbrush bristles can't quite get to, then it will likely turn into a cavity. A dentist can test to see if stain has become a cavity manually or with technology. To manually test requires the dentist to poke at it with a metal instrument (called an explorer); if the instrument sticks then it means the tooth has become soft, and the softness is a cavity. There are a couple of ways that technology can help as well. Various instruments like the DIAGNOdent can tell if the stain is a soft cavity or just hard tooth structure with stain.

If your dentist is both looking for a clinical stickiness and using dental technologies to look for a cavity, then I would wait until one of those two tests confirms decay. This is especially true if you are staying on top of your six-month cleanings. A cavity will not go from stain to a large cavity in just six months unless you have had previous head and neck radiation treatments that killed off your normal saliva flow. If avoiding cavities is your greatest concern and money is secondary, you could always get sealants and remove stain when present before placing the sealants.

Pain

You actually have a pretty good cavity indicator built into your body to let you know when you need a filling: PAIN! Pain is your body's way of telling you that there is something wrong and it needs to be fixed soon. You can get random pains that don't last long from things like popcorn kernels stuck in your gums or a sore tooth from grinding your teeth. You don't need to worry about those types of pain, but if the pain doesn't go away or goes away and returns in the same place, then you definitely have a problem that needs to be addressed. In this case, pain is actually your friend!

The tooth has several nerve fibers in it to sense pain. (See Chapter 8: Life Stages and Needed Dental Information for more information on the parts of the tooth and its development.) The center of each root has a hole where a blood vessel and nerve travel through. When the nerve reaches the crown portion of the tooth, the hole turns into a chamber. The nerve sends many small nerve fibers from that chamber into the dentin of the tooth. The outside 2 mm or so of the tooth is covered with enamel, which has no nerve fibers in it. When a cavity goes past the enamel and into the dentin, it will begin to elicit pain in those nerve fibers. You will know the cavity has gotten large enough that it definitely should be taken care of. If you let this pain continue, the cavity goes from just being a cavity to needing a root canal or extraction. Pain is your friend because it motivates you to not let a little problem turn into a big one.

If you let the pain continue for too long, the problem will perhaps go away and come back as an even worse problem. If that happens it means that the infection has completely destroyed the nerve. It won't start to hurt until you have an abscess. An abscess is where the infection has traveled through the hole that the nerve was in, all the way down the tooth and started to eat away at the bone. There are even cases of abscesses on upper teeth getting so big that they get into the brain and cause death. Not taking care of your teeth can actually kill you. Use your built-in safety nets of pain, and listen to your body to avoid little problems turning into big ones.

There are some minor dental problems that are better to take care of cheaply or even for free rather than paying for more costly dental treatments. One example is small chips in your back teeth. Often these can be smoothed out so they don't bother your tongue, instead of placing a filling. I am referring to instances when the missing tooth structure is about the size of a strawberry seed. Ask your dentist if he can just smooth out the area during your next exam. (This does not apply to large chips or fractures.) My office doesn't charge for little things like this. It is how we show our appreciation to our loyal patients.

Another problem that can often be repaired similarly would be chipped porcelain on crowns, especially crowns that are porcelain fused to metal. If a portion of the porcelain chips off, but doesn't break all the way through to tooth structure or in between two teeth causing food to get caught there, then it can be smoothed out. This often happens on crowns that are porcelain fused to metal instead of all porcelain because the bond between the porcelain and metal can be a weak point that allows the porcelain to chip off easily. The metal core underneath will protect the tooth from decay. Also, if the darkness of the metal is in an area that is not visible there is no need to replace the crown or bridge.

Just ask your dentist to smooth out the sharp edge of the porcelain and polish it. I've seen these easy fixes work over the last several years without any problems at all.

Habits

I'd like to end this chapter by discussing several slowly developing problems that turn into big problems over time. Most of these are bad habits of wear that will slowly do daily, undetectable damage to your teeth, and when continued for several years these bad habits can wear away 75% or more of your tooth structure. Once your tooth structure is gone, it can take a lot of time and money to get things back to where they once were. The best way to avoid paying unnecessary money is to avoid these habits or stop them if they are already happening.

The most common bad habit of tooth wear is also one of the most difficult to treat: bruxism. That term means grinding or squeezing the teeth together. It can be difficult to stop because you can't consciously stop during your sleep. Exact causes of nighttime bruxing are hard for science to figure out, but they are getting closer. Obstructive Sleep Apnea (OSA) is one of the known causes. Getting treated for OSA can stop your teeth wear. Daytime bruxing can also be hard to recognize if you are subconsciously doing it and it is not causing pain. If your teeth look like they have been worn, then discuss this tooth wear with your dentist. For more information on bruxism, see Chapter 6: Good Home Care to Avoid Extra Dental Visits.

Although not nearly as common as daytime and nighttime bruxing, you may create areas of significant dental wear from habits such as chewing your nails, biting thread or fishing line to cut it, or chewing a pen. Similarly, there are bad habits that cause chemical wear, such as sucking on acidic foods like lemons. If you are doing any of these wear-causing habits and brushing hard, then you will quickly get wear on the sides of your teeth as well. Some more bad habits that people consciously do are bulimia and excessive soda consumption. (See Chapter 6 for more information.) Both of these habits frequently bathe the teeth with large amounts of very strong acids.

If you know that you have any of these habits, work on stopping or replacing them with habits that won't wear down your teeth. I want to reiterate that these habits won't make a visible change from one day to another or even from one year to another; however, if continued over a decade, they can cause significant, irreversible wear that will make your smile look bad and your face look older. Ideally, when someone is talking or has their lips at rest you should see a little bit of their top teeth. As we age our skin sags and our upper lip covers more of our upper teeth even if they have no wear. When the teeth prematurely wear, it will cause the same look of no visible upper teeth when talking even in young people. If wear progresses to the point that the teeth can't be seen at rest, then a thirty-year-old can look like they have a seventy-year-old smile.

Finally, a quick, cheap, and easy way to save some money by avoiding unnecessary dental work is to make sure you don't keep your toothbrush for too long. Depending on the quality of your toothbrush and how hard you brush, getting a new one every six months may not be often enough. Once the bristles start to flare, they have lost their stiffness and won't brush food particles off of your teeth effectively. They will instead slide across the food particles, only removing the superficial layer. Spend a couple dollars on a new toothbrush that will do a good job of cleaning your teeth and you will save money down the road at the dental office. Instead of wasting the time you put into cleaning your teeth daily, use it effectively with a functional toothbrush.

Reading this book is a great way to get the knowledge you need to apply preventative measures and save you money. Your young-looking, money-saving, healthy smile will be a great reward for your proactive efforts!

Chapter 6

Good Home Care to Avoid Extra Dental Visits

Good home care is one of the easiest and cheapest ways to avoid spending extra money at the dental office. Again, the old adage, "An ounce of prevention is worth a pound of cure" is definitely sage advice. There are three solid legs that good home care stands on. They are proper brushing, flossing, and diet. I will go through each in detail and then add a few tips and tricks to save money and avoid losing more of your enamel.

Brushing

The first leg is brushing; for that to be a strong leg you need to brush for two minutes in the proper form. I remember learning in dental school that there was a study done where they put people in a room without a clock. They were told to brush for two minutes. The average time people brushed their teeth was 48 seconds. Like watching a pot of water boil, brushing can be boring and slow. People, especially kids, tend not to brush the full two minutes. A good way to make sure you are brushing for a full two minutes and evenly spreading 30 seconds to each quadrant is to get an electric toothbrush with a timer. This toothbrush, in my opinion, doesn't really do a significantly better job than a manual toothbrush (unless you have dexterity problems like severe arthritis), but its main benefit is that you keep brushing for the full two minutes.

When you skip out on any of those precious 120 seconds, you are not effectively brushing every surface of every tooth. Each tooth has at least three surfaces that should be brushed. The very back tooth in each of your four quadrants has four. The main three surfaces are tongue side, chewing surface, and cheek or lip side. The extra side on your back tooth is the back surface that faces your throat.

A common brushing error is to close your teeth and brush the cheek/lip surface only in the middle and not get up to the gums on the top or bottom teeth. Another error is skipping the area where you switch the angle of your brush. For example, right-handed people usually brush their front teeth and left side together, then rotate the brush 180 degrees to brush the right side. Often the area on the front right corner where they switch from the front teeth to the back right teeth gets skipped. The opposite is true for left-handed brushers. Finally, people often skip the tongue side of the back bottom teeth because it is a hard-to-get area. Unfortunately for your dentist, the hardest areas for you to get to are also the hardest areas for them to work on. People often skip these areas and get cavities in those places the most. Therefore getting your filling done won't be an easy or comfortable experience when you skip those areas. Dentistry would be so much easier if people would skip brushing their two front teeth and do an awesome job on the rest!

It is important to note that you shouldn't over brush. Brushing for too long or too hard (think massage, not scrub) can be detrimental to your enamel and your gums. If you over brush, it can lead to some bone loss. As the bone shrinks down away from the tooth, the gums follow. If that happens your smile won't look good, your teeth roots become exposed, and your teeth can be very sensitive. However, if you are going to error on one side, I'd probably suggest brushing too long. A little recession and keeping all your teeth seems better than losing them all to repetitive restorations and root canals. See Chapter 7: Common Dental

Problems and Solutions, for more information on dealing with sensitive teeth.

Flossing

The second leg to good home care is flossing. I embarrassingly found out in dental school that you have to floss more than just in between your teeth. You've never heard that either? Well, now you know you're not alone. I remember a professor who did exams on all incoming freshmen so that we could get approved for having good enough teeth to allow other students to work on us. The professor was looking around my mouth looking for cavities or other dental problems and noted the plaque and tartar buildup on the back of my back teeth. She said, "You need to start flossing behind your back teeth!" I remember thinking two things: "I look stupid right from the get go. Awesome!" and "What? Floss somewhere that isn't between two teeth?" Yes, that is right, your toothbrush can't quite reach back there and you'll start to build up tartar near your gums.

Besides flossing in between all your teeth and behind your back ones, you also need to floss correctly. Going straight in and out is definitely better than doing nothing at all, but it doesn't quite get everything. To floss correctly you need to curve your floss around the tooth. Think of making each side of your floss into adorable little arms that want to hug your tooth. Slide the hugging floss up and down one tooth. Then hug the other tooth and slide up and down that one as well. Repeat this for every set of touching teeth and behind the last one in each quadrant.

I often get asked, "Is it better to floss first then brush or brush first then floss." Honestly, like many people, I hate flossing and have a better solution, but first I will answer this question. Have you ever smelled the floss after you floss with it, especially if it has been a couple of days since you last flossed? It can smell like the bottom of your boot after stepping in swamp mud. Not good! Therefore, I think it is better to floss first, then brush second to avoid the bad breath you would get from flossing decaying food in your teeth. There is logic in the opposite though. If you brush first and then floss, then you remove a lot of the food from brushing so the floss can do a better job by only working on what is left. Ideally, I recommend brushing, flossing, and finishing with a nice rinse of something like Listerine. That way you rinse the swamp mud away and don't knock over the next person you talk to.

Like I mentioned before, I am a dentist that hates flossing just like most of you. At least I'm honest. I get around it by using an amazing device called a Waterpik. I love this little machine. (The cordless ones usually don't work near as well as the plug-in kind.) I'm hooked on it because I think you can use it instead of floss, while not having to worry about leaving some swamp mud in your mouth. Also, I think it does a better job than flossing does. I've tested it several times when I've flossed and then used a Waterpik. I definitely see little bits of food get flushed out that the floss didn't catch. I've flipped the experiment around and when flossing after the Waterpik, I do not find any remaining food particles.

For those with Obsessive Compulsive Disorder, I need to put a little check and balance in here. Don't create a new daily oral hygiene routine of brushing, flossing, "waterpicking," and Listerine rinsing after every meal and when you go to bed. That would be way too much. Go out and spend time with your children. If you don't have any children, go save some baby seals. Either way, you'll get a lot more out of life by not going overboard on your oral hygiene. Brushing twice a day for two minutes and flossing (or "waterpicking") daily will take care of your mouth for most people with a decent diet.

Diet

Speaking of diet, it is the third leg of our stool. If you take meticulous care of your teeth yet have a horrible diet, you'll still have numerous dental problems. On the other hand, if you have an amazing diet and slack in your home care, then you won't have as many problems with your teeth. Basically, this is the most important leg of the stool. Understanding what makes for a good or bad diet will help you save time and money at the dental office.

What constitutes a good diet in relation to your teeth? Most importantly, simple sugars are very bad. Complex carbohydrates are kind of bad. Sticky and acidic things are bad too. Other than that, it doesn't make a huge difference what you eat or drink. Your body needs a lot more complexity of guidelines on what to eat when it comes to proper nutrition, but your teeth are fairly simple. So, let's break these things down into more detail.

What is the difference between a simple sugar and complex carbohydrate? An easy way to understand the difference is to think of sweet foods versus starchy foods. Simple sugars are sweet like fruit, table sugar, honey, juice, candy, etc. Complex carbohydrates are starchy like potatoes, bread, whole wheat pasta, etc. The more simple the sugar, the easier it is for the bacteria in your mouth to digest it. The easier it is to digest, the faster the bacteria can create cavities. See Chapter 7: Common Dental Problems and Solutions for a more detailed explanation on cavities and how they are formed.

The stickier the carbohydrate (simple or complex), the more likely it is to cause cavities. For example, raisins and crackers both tend to stick into the grooves and spaces in between your teeth. The longer these food particles hang around, the more time the bacteria has to digest the sugars and produce acids. You can probably see why candy is so bad. It is usually made of very simple sugars and sticky ingredients. A double whammy!

It is important to note here while talking about stickiness that the amount of sugar isn't as bad as how long it is on your teeth. There is an example I frequently share that gets the point across well. Imagine person A; she drinks a six-pack of soda every day, three cans at lunch and three cans at dinner. Imagine person B; he drinks only one can of the same soda, but he drinks it slowly throughout the day at his desk. Which person is going to get more cavities? If you guessed A because she bathed her teeth in six times as much sugar you would be wrong. The effect of slowly drinking one can of soda throughout the day gives the bacteria in your mouth a continuous supply of sugar to grow on your teeth. It is like giving steroids to the bacteria. The cavities grow huge and quickly. Person A quickly pushed most of that sugar past the bacteria in her mouth and into her stomach. Her cavities might not be getting huge, but her belly probably is. The benefit for Person A is that you can always exercise off the fat, but Person B can't grow back the enamel.

Finally, the more acidic your food is, the worse it is for your teeth. Not only does acid make the environment of your mouth more hospitable to the bacteria and cause cavities by producing acid, the increase in acidity can dissolve your teeth. Sucking lemons is an example of a very acidic habit. When the acidity gets bad enough, it will dissolve the enamel off of your teeth. Even worse is a little bit of acidity combined with abrasion. For example, sucking on a lemon for a short time will bathe your teeth with acid, which will dissolve the outer layer of enamel. Then, if you brush quickly after the lemon-flavored acid bath, you'll wear away the decalcified organic matrix (non-dissolvable parts of the tooth) that the enamel sits in, losing that tooth structure forever!

Bad Habits

Along those lines, whenever we eat, the acidity drops in our mouth. For that reason it actually isn't a good idea to brush immediately after eating. Waiting ten minutes after a normal meal will allow our mouth's acidity to return to normal and even allow the calcium to soak back up. Brushing immediately will wear away that matrix, which speeds up premature wearing of the teeth. This is especially important if you have slight acid reflux during the night. Waiting a little bit before brushing when you wake up will allow the recalcification of your teeth and decrease the amount of wear that happens over time.

There are a myriad of other problems that can contribute to premature tooth wear. Some of the most common are chewing ice, biting your fingernails, and biting on a pen. Teeth were made for chewing food and believe it or not, your teeth hardly touch while chewing food. Once they do touch when chewing, it triggers swallowing. All the chewing before that keeps the food in between your teeth so that they don't quite touch. The above habits will add massive amounts of contact and wear to your teeth causing them to age very fast. By the way, this is a good trick for swallowing pills when you have a hard time doing it. Put the pill in your mouth, touch your teeth together, and then try to swallow. The touching of the teeth will trigger the swallowing reflex and make it easier!

The fastest way to wear down teeth is through strong acid as just described, but the second fastest way is through bruxism. That is from grinding teeth, clenching, or a combination of both. Collectively, these problems along with other Temporomandibular Joint (TMJ) problems are called Temporomandibular Joint Disorder (TMD). Let me take a minute to note a couple of things. The problem is not called TMJ; that is a common misnomer of the public. TMJ is the joint, whereas TMD is the dysfunction of that joint. Also, there has been a lot of research done on TMD in the last few years that has changed some long-held beliefs. Unless your dentist has taken specific classes on TMD, they likely will not know very much about the current research showing that TMD, especially nighttime bruxism, is caused less from your teeth (occlusion) and more from your central nervous system.

If bruxism is causing excessive wear or pain, definitely see someone who has up-to-date training on the subject. If you have mild wear, abfractions, recession, etc., then evaluate the following tests to see if there are some easy fixes that might resolve your problems. As always, if your minor problem isn't fixed, then go see someone with training who can help you with such a complex issue. Are you waking up in the morning with soreness in your teeth, jaw, or head? You may be bruxing, even if you don't have pain. A good test to determine if you are bruxing is to move your jaw out and to one side, right when you wake up. Does your jaw quiver? If so, your muscles are fatigued from overuse during the night. This means you are bruxing and should seek help. If your jaw isn't fatigued in the morning, are you doing it during the day at all? Most people who are daytime bruxing are actually not aware of it. I often tell people that they have significant wear signs on their teeth and they tell me, "That can't be possible, I don't grind my teeth." Though I never do, I want to ask, "Then who is sedating you and taking sandpaper or a grinder to your teeth?"

Daytime bruxism often happens when you are "zoning out" of the real world like driving your commute on autopilot, surfing the web, or reading a book. To become consciously aware if you are bruxing, try the following test. Set an alarm on your phone to go off every ten to fifteen minutes on your commute or while you are reading. When it goes off, notice immediately what you were doing with your teeth. How do they feel? Were you squeezing them together? Do they feel slightly sore? If any type of bruxism was happening, you are now aware of it! Realizing you are daytime bruxing is half the battle. Now you can recognize when you are doing it and work on breaking that habit. During those times that you find yourself bruxing, periodically take a breath and blow air out of your relaxed mouth. The position your jaw is in when you finish blowing out the air is the most natural and relaxed position for your TMJ. Try to keep it in that position without touching your teeth together.

The above habit of bruxing is an example of a bad habit. In addition to brushing, flossing, and a good diet, there is another good habit that can help you avoid extra visits to the dental office: the proper use of fluoride. You may have heard some bad things about fluoride. Many of those misconceptions and a detailed explanation of the benefits of fluoride for all ages can be found in Chapter 10: Common Misconceptions. Basically, taking fluoride pills or drops until about age nine will help to strengthen the developing teeth in the bone. Additionally, if you are cavity prone or have tooth sensitivity, using a fluoride rinse and definitely using toothpaste with fluoride in it will help strengthen the teeth that are already grown in.

Use the information in this chapter to take your home care to a new level. Keep your teeth looking great, feeling great, and problem free!

Chapter 7

Common Dental Problems and Solutions

This chapter focuses on several common problems and their best solutions so that you know if the solution is something you can do at home or if you need a visit to the dental office. As always, if you have severe pain, go to your dentist. Likewise, if the pain doesn't improve, then go to your dentist. If you have any significant medical problems, then see your physician. Don't avoid taking care of a small problem—they often turn into larger ones!

What's the most common dental pain? A sore tooth obviously! There can be a myriad of different causes. The following are the most likely diagnoses from the correlated symptoms of a sore tooth or teeth:

1. Does it hurt mostly when you bite? If no, skip to paragraph #3. If yes, Does it hurt more when you bite down or when you let go? If it hurts more to bite down than let go, then keep reading. If it is the latter, skip to paragraph #2. This biting pain can be caused by a lot of different things. If this pain is mostly present in the morning, then it is most likely due to clenching or grinding during the night. This can happen from daytime clenching as well. Basically, if the tooth only hurts when you bite on it and not the rest of the time, then it is probably due to some

sort of clenching or grinding. See if you can recognize when you might be grinding your teeth and then try to stop it. Take some ibuprofen, and if the pain subsides in forty-eight hours, you should be fine. If the pain doesn't get better or especially if it gets worse, then go see your dentist to see if there is another problem. Bruxing not only wears teeth down, but even if you don't slide your teeth across each other it can cause a lot of problems. Teeth interdigitate when you bite down. That means that any one tooth usually is hitting against two opposing teeth. If you kick your jaw out to the side a little and squeeze that can often make a single tooth hit against two opposing teeth. The two opposing teeth will each take 50% of the force and the tooth hitting against them takes 100% of the opposing force. That causes some temporary damage to the bone around the tooth, which results in pretty bad pain. If the clenching or grinding stops, then the pain usually resolves in forty-eight hours or less.

2. You probably have cracked tooth syndrome. This most often happens when you have a silver filling in a tooth for a long period of time that is fairly large. The metal expands more than the tooth when it gets hot and causes the tooth to slowly crack over time. When the crack gets big enough that it allows for a lot of bending, then it can start to hurt. Don't wait too long to get this fixed because it can go from just a crown (the normal way to fix it) to needing a root canal or even an extraction. A crown usually fixes the problem because it makes the whole biting surface a single, uniform material so that you can't push one cusp away from the other.

3. Does cold air make your tooth hurt? If the answer is no, skip to paragraph #4. Cold air sensitivity is most commonly caused by recession. This originally was thought to be a result of brushing too hard on your gums. It turns

out it is most commonly due to clenching and/or grinding. This causes your teeth to slightly flex in the middle and that leads to bone loss and notches being formed in the side of your tooth next to the gums. As the bone recedes, the gums follow and the root becomes exposed. The root has nerve endings that go out to the surface whereas the crown portion of the tooth does not. There are no nerves in the enamel. These exposed nerves in the root can be sensitive to temperature and sometimes to touch (like a toothbrush or a fingernail scratching the area). The best way to take care of this problem once recession has occurred is to use toothpaste intended for teeth sensitivity. Brushing with it helps a little, but even better is to cover the sensitive area with a film of the toothpaste and let that sit there. Do that both morning and night when you brush. The longer it sits on there, the more it will be absorbed into the tooth and protect you from sensitivity. If that doesn't help, then there could be other problems or you may need a more severe protection of the root surface. You can get fillings to cover the notch in the side of the tooth or the exposed root. Fillings help protect against sensitivity, and it is harder than the root surface so natural wear from toothbrush abrasion and acidic chemicals wear on the filling rather than the soft inside of your tooth. You can also get fluoride treatments that help with sensitivity. Again, if these treatments aren't helping, then you could have various problems that require a filling or root canal. Don't go more than two weeks trying to make it get better without getting results. If things get worse or stay the same for two weeks, definitely go see your dentist.

4. Does cold make your tooth feel better? If no, skip to paragraph #5. This almost always means that you need a root canal. The cold causes the inflammation and swelling to

reduce and take pressure off the nerve. Pretty much the only way to fix that problem is to get a root canal. Don't be afraid, even though root canals have a bad reputation. The procedure itself usually isn't that bad. It is the pain that makes you need the root canal that is bad. The root canal takes about an hour and gets rid of the pain!

5. We've ruled out biting pain or cold being the source of your pain. Does your tooth hurt to sweets? If not, skip to paragraph #6. This has two primary causes. The bacteria that cause cavities live off sugar. When you give them some it can irritate the tooth they are burrowing a hole into. It can also be from recession as stated in paragraph #3 like cold can do. Try the suggestions described in that paragraph, and if they don't get better in two weeks or get worse, go see your dentist. You probably have a cavity and not just recession.

6. Does your tooth hurt periodically without any stimulation? If you have ruled out pain from clenching and grinding, this is likely due to a few things. Most of these problems require that you see a dentist, especially the first time.

   a. **Cavity:** This can cause a tooth to hurt randomly. If the pain is dull and achy, you likely have a deep cavity that is closer to the nerve. Pain is your body's way of telling you to get it taken care of. If it is sharp, especially if it wakes you up at night, then you are probably past the point of no return and you need a root canal.

   b. **Abscess:** This is when the bacteria from a cavity reach a hole in the middle of the tooth where the main nerve body travels. The bacteria then travel down this tunnel to your bone and begin to infect your bone. It isn't always visible on an x-ray. It only will be when the infection has eaten away a large enough amount of bone to be visible, and it always requires a root canal. Unfortunately, sometimes this can happen after you have already had a root canal; it is known as a failed root canal, and it needs to be retreated.

c. **Allergy or other sinus problems:** Every spring when the pollen begins to float around, there is a spike in people coming to my office afraid they might need a root canal. The nerves from your upper teeth travel near the maxillary sinus, and sometimes your brain can interpret the irritation in that area as coming from your teeth. Take something that will subside the allergy symptoms and see if it goes away in a few days. If not, get checked by your dentist.

d. **Referred pain:** Sometimes the pain is a referred pain and you don't have any problem in the area that hurts. The pain is being caused by a source in another area. This pain is often due to something "upstream" like your neck muscles. One patient underwent two root canals and eventual extractions of the "painful" teeth since the pain didn't go away. The source of the pain wasn't from the teeth sadly, but a referred pain from her neck muscles. The neck was postured forward, and the muscles had to overwork to hold the neck up in that position. Her neck was postured forward because she had lower back pain that made her move her back forward to keep the pain down. She only needed to resolve the lower back pain to improve her back position; her neck muscles could then be used normally and not hurt or cause referred pain to the area of her teeth. Instances of referred pain can be complicated to figure out at times, so it can be beneficial to see a physical therapist for proper diagnosis.

What about sores or soreness in the mouth that isn't felt in a tooth? There are hundreds of different problems that could be causing pain in the soft tissues of your mouth—anything from the common Aphthous Ulcer (canker sore) to a localized case of periodontal disease. The good news is the two most common periodic sores in the mouth (Aphthous Ulcer and Herpetic Lesion) both have medicines that make dealing with them much easier.

An Aphthous Ulcer is commonly known as a canker sore. It is a sore that develops when something triggers your body to start a localized autoimmune response. Basically, it is your body attacking itself in that one spot. They can be very painful too! The best way to stop a canker sore is to get a prescription that has a topical anesthetic to numb the area as well as a topical steroid to stop the autoimmune response. This makes it much more comfortable and speeds up the healing process. There are different kinds of steroids; this type will not make you grow more facial hair, get a deeper voice, or have bigger muscles. The lesion can be stimulated by many different things such as trauma (banging an area of the mouth with a toothbrush) or foods (often hyperallergenic foods such as nuts). Avoiding whatever stimuli that triggers them can help reduce the frequency in which they occur. You can also see your physician or dentist for a prescription.

A Herpetic Lesion (commonly called a cold sore) usually appears on the lower lip. It is from the Herpes Virus, and although that sounds terrible, at least 60% of adults have come in contact with this virus. It is not usually the same virus as genital herpes. The lesion is often preceded by a tingly sensation in the lip where the lesion will appear. If you take an antiviral at this point, it will significantly decrease the size and duration of the lesion. Once the lesion has appeared a couple of times, you will get a good idea of what those precursor symptoms feel like and be able to reduce the overall symptoms greatly with the proper medication. See your physician or dentist for a prescription.

Another common sore or pain in the mouth that isn't always felt in the teeth is an abscess. An abscess is an infection around a tooth root in the bone. It is most often from a cavity that got so large the bacteria reached the hole in the middle of the tooth where the main nerve and blood vessel travel. This allows the bacteria to travel down easily into the bone at the tip of the root. The bacteria eat away at the bone creating a pocket of infection. Sometimes it will burrow its way out the side of the bone where a pimple-like bump will appear. This relieves the pressure to and can often mark a change from very painful to not too tender. The swelling will sometimes cause a bulging on the side of your face that will hurt when your teeth are without pain. You will likely need either an extraction or a root canal. If you don't do anything it will cycle back and forth between very painful and normal. See your dentist as soon as possible to get the infection under control and eliminated.

Finally, the other very common non-tooth pain in the mouth is having something stuck in your gums. In my experience, the two most common pieces of food are popcorn kernels or apple skins. These pieces of food will often slowly dissolve over a couple of days and then stop hurting. A related problem happens if you have a small gap between two teeth. If that gap is big enough so floss doesn't "snap" when used, yet smaller than 2 mm, it will be a food trap. All types of food can get stuck and cause pain. This often happens if a filling chips or breaks off a small portion in between it and another tooth. The more hard and fibrous a food is, the more it will stick in places like this and hurt. Meats are the biggest source of impacted food, and harder meats like jerky can be especially painful. Floss might not always get the stuck food out very well; you may need to get the space closed with a new filling or orthodontics. One way to get the stuck food out is to tie a knot in the floss so that there is a little bump or ball in the floss. Pull this through sideways and it will help pull out the stuck food. It is even better to get a Waterpik and flush the area thoroughly.

If you have one of the lesser common, yet hundreds of other types of sores in the mouth, it is best to see your dentist for further evaluation (especially if the sore or lesion doesn't go away in two weeks). Get evaluated soon so that you can get proper treatment and keep it from turning into a bigger problem. Even if it may be scary to find out what the problem could be, it is always better to know and get treated than to allow it to get worse.

Other Dental Problems

Halitosis

People often come to the dental office with the concern of bad breath (halitosis). Like most other issues in the mouth, there can be several causes. If you are brushing and flossing your teeth regularly and getting regular cleanings, then bad breath is probably not from your gums. Bad cavities, especially ones under crowns, can cause halitosis. Those would need an exam and x-rays to diagnose. If there are no signs of decay, then you need to move to the back of the mouth. Is there a large buildup of gunk on the back of your tongue? You can get a tongue scraper to scrape off buildup, which is caused especially when you are sick. Regular tongue cleaning can be a very good thing. You should do it every time you brush your teeth. If that doesn't help, then you could have anything from post-nasal drip to acid reflux. It would be good to see an Ear, Nose, and Throat specialist or at least your general physician for recommendations on what to do.

What can you do for periodic, short-term bad breath? Like I stated earlier, daily brushing, flossing, and occasional posterior tongue cleaning can keep the majority of bad bacteria down. What if you are headed out on a date and need to make sure everything is good? Definitely use an alcohol-based mouth rinse. Scope, for example, is not a good option; it just makes your breath smell good by covering anything up. On the other hand, Listerine will kill some of the halitosis-causing bacteria and keep your breath better for longer. Chewing gum can help because it keeps saliva moving in your mouth, which keeps things fresh as well.

Painful Dental Work

Pain after getting dental work done is often something that makes people wonder if they should go into the dental office or not. It is common to have some sensitivity in your tooth and gums after a filling, especially if the dentist told you it was a large filling. If you do, an anti-inflammatory like ibuprofen is the best thing to take. Tylenol just works on the brain and not the source of pain, so it isn't as good. If you feel like you are contacting more on the new restoration when chewing then definitely call your dentist to get that adjusted, especially if it is made of porcelain or metal instead of composite. Sometimes the bonding agent (what the dentist rubs onto your tooth before placing the filling) can create a thin film on the tooth and teeth around it that wears off in a day or two. If it doesn't get better in a couple of days, then definitely get in for an adjustment.

Getting a filling to the perfect size is hard to do without over adjusting it. If your dentist is trying to not over adjust and get it just right, you will occasionally be left you with too big of a filling. This adjustment should be done at no charge to you as a follow-up to the actual restoration. If the doctor told you that you had a very deep cavity that means it got very close to the nerve. Also, if you were having pain in the tooth before the filling was done, it can stay painful afterward. If that pain is from the nerve, as often happens in deep fillings or previously hurting teeth, it can take a long time for the nerve to heal. I usually tell a patient that if it hurts unbearably bad or is not getting better fast enough, then we can do a root canal. If it is getting better, even very slowly, and they can wait, then I would wait to avoid the root canal. Sometimes a sensitive nerve can get traumatized again and require a root canal, so be sure to take care of it while it is healing by avoiding extreme temperatures or pressures. My wife had a similar situation with her tooth; she kept getting hit in the chin by our children as they would stand up in her lap. Sometimes even kids can cause a root canal!

Flossing Problems

Other post-treatment dental problems can be irritating. Is it hard to get floss in between your teeth now? Is it too easy and you get food stuck in between your teeth? Both of those flossing problems should have you go back to your dentist to get them fixed, as they will not take care of themselves. Is your filling rough? Wait a few days and see if it smooths out. Sometimes the roughness is from the bonding agent, but it wears off easily. If a week has gone by and it still bugs you, then get in for a quick polishing of the restoration.

Dark Spots

One problem that often brings people into the dental office is a dark spot on a filling. It can be hard to know if this is a cavity or not. Sometimes it is just the metal edge of a porcelain fused to metal crown. The metal used to be covered by the gums, but now that they have receded it is visible. Sometimes it is from a filling having its edge (margin) debond, which allows liquid to sit in between it and the tooth, soak in, and eventually cause a dark stain. Sometimes it is a cavity. Sometimes the open margin that allows for a stain also allows for bacteria, which turns into a cavity. It can also be the start of a cavity that re-calcifies and becomes what we call "arrested," meaning the cavity has stopped and isn't progressing anymore. It can be hard to differentiate between all of these options, so you should get it examined during your next cleaning. Consider scheduling an exam now to get it evaluated if your next check-up isn't for a while. If you are experiencing pain in the tooth with the dark spot, then definitely get in soon so you don't go from needing a cavity to needing a root canal and a crown. Your pocketbook will thank you!

Chapter 8

Life Stages and Needed Dental Information

Our dental needs change as we progress through various stages of life. This chapter will go through each stage and explain what is happening to you and what things you should focus on to have optimal dental health. As an additional resource, there are tooth loss and tooth development charts in the appendix.

Prenatal

We start developing our teeth while in the womb and children even periodically are born with one or more of their primary teeth already erupted. Talk about a recipe for painful feedings! Everyone's teeth start developing in the womb. Illnesses, trauma, and excessive stress can cause bad tooth formations, especially in the enamel. Typically, the first tooth starts to form during the fourth month of pregnancy. That means when your baby bump is starting to be noticeable to other people, your little one is starting to grow a tooth. Because teeth start forming during pregnancy, it is important for the mother to get prenatal vitamins before pregnancy and proper nutrition before, during, and after pregnancy. (See Chapter 10: Common Misconceptions for more information on fluoride.)

Newborn

If you haven't started doing prenatal fluoride (which is OK, it's understandable why you would want to limit any chemical intake during fetal development), now can be a good time to start. The average age at which a baby's first set of upper front teeth finish forming is at one and a half months old. In other words, after two months babies have already passed the time when any ingested fluoride is going to help their teeth. The baby molars finish forming before their first birthday. So, if you've waited until your baby's first birthday to start fluoride it will only help the adult teeth, and not even all of them. For example, the first molars are usually about halfway done forming the crown around age one. Cavities usually form in between teeth and in the chewing surfaces. Therefore, half of the likely cavity areas on that tooth have already formed and ingesting fluoride won't help them. (See Chapter 10 for more information on fluoride.)

One big question parents of newborns have for the dentist is whether or not it is acceptable for their children to suck their thumb or on a pacifier. There are a lot of different opinions on this subject from dentists and orthodontists. I will give you my own opinions and the logic behind them so you can make an informed decision for yourself. There are some bad things that can happen if children suck on their finger(s) or a pacifier for too long or too hard. It can push the palate forward and cause a deformation of the bone. This can lead to speech, swallowing, and aesthetic problems that can be difficult to fix later on. Research shows that in most cases, if the child stops by the age of three, the pressure from the lips will pull the teeth back into the proper position. Teeth are in an equilibrium position that is the happy medium between the tongue pressure out and the lips or cheek pressure in. As long as that pressure isn't too strong from things like thumb sucking or poor swallowing technique, then the teeth are more likely to be in a good position.

Some orthodontists recommend to just wait for children to go to school, and they will stop from peer pressure or on their own. I don't agree with this for two reasons. First, I don't want to allow a shaming situation to happen to my child if I can help to avoid it. Secondly, although it can be fixed, it is usually more complicated. I'd rather do it naturally when it is easier and cheaper. So, if your kid is thumb-sucking or using a pacifier at the age of three, how do you get them to stop? This can be a complicated answer as it depends greatly on the child and when they do it. The hardest part of the habit to stop is when it is subconsciously happening at night. Even children who want to stop the habit may continue to do it because they are doing it without thinking while sleeping. Positive rewards for reaching goals of diminished use tend to work best, but when children continue the habit without thinking at night you have another good option, and it's cheap too!

You can build a homemade anti-digit (meaning finger) sucking device. Go to your hardware store and buy a couple PVC pipe end caps that will fit over your child's finger(s) without being too big. Drill two holes in the side of the end caps. Take some string and tie a knot in one end and feed it through one of the holes. Do the same thing for the other side. Now slide this over the desired finger(s) and tie it into place around the wrist without being too tight. This will usually work well to get them out of the habit because they won't want to suck on the PVC and taking it off usually requires two hands. The hand that the device is on will not be able to reach the knot on the wrist and untie it. They can use their teeth if they are really motivated, but it works pretty well during the night. If they still untie it at night, you can tie knots that can only be cut and replace the strings each day until they break the habit.

Toddler

Your child will continue to have teeth erupt until about the age of two. They tend to get their first baby (primary) molars around eighteen months and the second set comes a little after the age of two. See the Eruption, Calcification, and Exfoliation charts in the appendix for more detailed information and as a quick reference. I see a lot of toddlers in my dental practice, and it is usually because of trauma. These little ones are exploring the world, trying to crawl on things around the house, and learning to walk. All of which can be a painful learning experience. They also don't know how to put their hands out as they fall; thus they tend to "soften" the blow with their head most of the time. This often chips front teeth or tears tissue.

My second son, for example, was an aggressive learner and was able to walk at nine months. He didn't quite have the coordination to walk well and kept falling into things and catching his lip on them. He tore the tissue where the lip attaches to the face on the inside; we could lift his lip and see into the bone. I was fresh out of dental school and didn't have much trauma training yet, so we took him to the physician. We were told that they don't often place stitches even in cases like that. They just recommend helping the kid avoid more falls and letting it repair itself naturally unless an infection sets in. Most parents dislike hearing that there isn't a lot you can do with these chips, bruises, and tears. Teeth often bite through lips and the tongue. The good news is that they heal quickly and eventually children will lose these "practice teeth" anyway. In situations where extractions do need to occur, just remember that around the age of six the child will start to get the toothy grin back.

Furthermore, when it comes to smiles, many parents wonder if having spaces between the teeth is bad. Other than having baby-model smiles, spaces (diastemas) are actually good for two reasons. The first is that when the teeth aren't touching they are less likely to get a cavity (unless they are just barely spaced enough for food to get stuck instead of pass through). Also, children are less likely to have crowding later on when their adult teeth erupt.

Even with spaces it is still possible to get cavities. Although I rarely see it because parents are much more educated about children's teeth now than they used to be. Sometimes one-year-old babies will get bad cavities in between their upper two front teeth. It is so sad to see such small children have cavities. This usually happens because the parents are giving their child a juice that has a large amount of sugar (usually high-fructose corn syrup). Furthermore, the problem is exacerbated when children are allowed to slowly sip juice throughout the day or night. Like I said, most parents know this is bad and don't let their kids do it.

The problems associated with children drinking sugary juice can also happen as kids get older and move on to a sippy cup. The problem with sippy cups is that the children keep it with them and slowly sip it throughout the day. If you are only letting your child use it to be spill proof and drink at mealtimes, then it usually won't be a problem. Similarly, many parents ask if it is OK to put a child to bed with a bottle. In regards to cavities, children will be fine if they quickly drink the bottle (as long as it isn't a sugary juice) and fall asleep. If they drink a little then keep sipping on it throughout the night, then they will get cavities.

So, when should you first take your child to the dentist to see if they have cavities? The American Academy of Pediatric Dentistry and the American Academy of Pediatrics both recommend that your child be seen by the age of one. This is mainly to verify that there are no dental malformations or early incidence of tooth decay. It is also so that you as a parent can be educated about issues that we are discussing in this chapter and throughout the book.

What should you expect during those first few visits? At that first one-year visit expect to get a quick exam and basically just have your questions answered. Also, your dentist or hygienist will probably recommend you start your child on fluoride if the water isn't fluoridated where you live. Children are probably going to resist anyone taking a look inside their mouth. That brings me to an important point for children in the dental office. It is my opinion that you should never force anything traumatic on a child without their permission except in cases of advanced or extreme cavities where the parents won't allow sedation. Those traumatic experiences often stick with them the rest of their lives. I've had very capable adults shake in fear when they get a cleaning. They say and know that nothing painful will happen during the cleaning, but they still have an extreme fear in the dental chair. Again, these are very successful and capable people. The amygdala in the limbic system of our brain can remember fear for a long time and in powerful ways that is hard to overcome.

For that reason I only force things that won't be traumatic on children, such as a quick exam on a one-year-old. Then we follow it up with something positive. Children feel me pull their lips back or even slightly open their teeth, but after a couple seconds of looking it's over and done. They realize that nothing hurt, and they get a toy for their participation. This has been very beneficial for toddlers in my practice. If a child does need something traumatic like a needle and fillings, yet they absolutely don't want to participate, I feel it is better to partially or fully sedate children. It can also be a good option to wait a year or so if the cavity is small enough. One year can make a significant difference in temperament and cooperation.

As you build these positive experiences, we hope to have the child sit down in the chair and do quick and simple cleanings and exams. Then by age five we hope to get full exams and cleanings. When this sequence is followed, children often do very well and look forward to their dental visits! Positive dental visits also help in creating desire to cooperate with daily home dental care.

Child

One of the biggest life events for children is losing their first tooth. It is the passage from little kid to big kid years. To top it all off, a fairy brings you free money! When does this typically happen? As long as children learn to put their hands out when they fall, then teeth typically fall out around age six. It is most commonly one of the two lower central incisors (front two middle teeth on the bottom). Sometimes it is the upper centrals, but not as often. It can often happen as early as age five or as late as age seven. In my experience kids that get their baby teeth in early also tend to lose them earlier and get their adult teeth early too.

There are a few generalities that are easy to remember and help parents have less anxiety about what is happening to their children's teeth. Kids usually start losing teeth at age six and lose all eight front teeth during the next two years. Then, they take a break for two years from ages eight to ten and start losing the rest during years ten to twelve. Think age 6–8 losing, 8–10 resting, 10–12 losing again. They get their first permanent molars at the start of losing teeth and therefore are often called six-year-old molars. They get their next permanent molars at the finish and are often called twelve-year-old molars. There is another set of molars called wisdom teeth, but we will discuss them in a later section.

Be aware that when six-year-old molars come in (first adult molars), they don't often hurt and can sneak in without you or your child knowing it. This creates a problem because as molars poke through the gums, they sit right at gum level. Their rough surface with its grooves and fissures often catches a lot of food. Your child isn't used to brushing behind their second primary molar since they've been brushing that way for a few years. In this situation the new molar doesn't get touched. They come in for their regular check-up at six and a half and all of the sudden they have a cavity on a permanent tooth! It is a very sad situation that I'd like to see never happen. To avoid this, just periodically check behind the second molar starting at about age five-and-a-half. Once you see those molars start to poke through, tell your child to brush back there every time they brush. Eventually the molars will erupt enough that it will be natural to brush and keep clean like the other teeth.

Besides fluoride and good home care there is something you can do to help your child have fewer cavities on these molars. Especially at this age when they aren't self-motivated to take care of their teeth. That extra something is placing sealants. Sealants are like fillings that start out extra liquidy and are usually only placed on molars. They help because the grooves in molars often get too skinny and deep for the toothbrush bristles to properly reach and clean out. When this happens, food will sit on the molar and allow bacteria to grow and eat away at the tooth undisturbed. It is always sad to see a seven-year-old have a large cavity on an adult molar when they are so brand new. To do the sealant, the dental office will clean the grooves and place a filling that starts out liquid. It will flow into those grooves. They shine a light on the liquid filling to turn the liquid hard, which makes teeth easier to clean.

Preteen

In the previous section we already discussed when children lose their teeth and how children generally take a break from losing teeth between ages eight and ten. This is unfortunately referred to as the "ugly duckling" stage. There are two reasons why this makes your child's smile look a little funny. First, your children have these huge, adult-sized teeth in their child-sized bodies. The second is that the adult teeth tend to be more yellow than the primary teeth. This yellow color looks worse at this time because it is contrasting against the primary canines that are very white. Once the remaining primary teeth fall out and the child has only adult teeth, the contrast is gone and the teeth don't look so terribly yellow anymore.

This is a good age to be evaluated for braces. Most orthodontists don't want to start intervention until all eight front teeth are in. Even so, at that point they usually only want to use space maintainers when severe crowding or narrow arches are present (often caused from excessive finger sucking discussed earlier in this chapter). It is always good to get a consult from an orthodontist if you and your dentist are not sure what should be done. Fortunately, exams are usually free, and the worst thing that will happen is that they will tell you it is too early and to return in a few years.

There are two primary reasons why braces are needed. The first is just to make your child's smile look perfect. It has become normal for children to get braces and have straight teeth. If children do have crooked teeth and don't get them straightened, it can look abnormal despite it being the way most people naturally look without orthodontic help. It is funny to me to see kids ask for braces even when they have straight teeth because they don't want to feel "left out." Gone are the days of being called "brace face" or "metal mouth." The second reason why braces are done is for various misalignments that are severe enough to cause problems down the road. I won't cover those problems here, but there are definitely cases where getting braces will help more than just to give you a pretty smile.

Teen

The teen years usually start after all adult teeth have come in (except wisdom teeth). The wisdom teeth can come in as early as age fifteen, but for most people wisdom teeth start to show around age eighteen to twenty. Most people don't have enough room for their wisdom teeth to fully erupt in the mouth; thus, they are often extracted during the teen years. Even if you do have enough room, wisdom teeth don't do anything beneficial. Most of our chewing happens on the second premolar and the first molar. I tell people that if their wisdom teeth come in fully like a normal tooth, then they won't receive any pressure from me to get them out. Likewise if they stay down in the bone and don't partially erupt, it is OK not to extract. If they only partially erupt, then I say it is much better to remove them. Problems can ensue if a portion of the tooth sticks out of the gums or even bumps up against the crown of the tooth in front of it. Because gums don't attach to enamel, a pocket around the unerupted part of the crown will be created. Bacteria will get into that pocket from the portion of the tooth that pokes through the gingiva or bumps up against the tooth in front of it. There isn't much you can do to keep bacteria from getting out of control; infections or cavities below the gums will likely ensue. This is why your dentist encourages that your wisdom teeth be extracted.

Since wisdom teeth are hard to clean, they often get cavities when they fully erupt. When this happens, I give my patients the option of doing the filling to fix the cavity or getting them extracted. As long as they are aware of their options I let them choose and then help their choice turn out the best for them. The younger you are when you get the extractions done the less traumatic it is. It is best to have them extracted when the root is about one-third of its full length. This makes the roots long enough so that the crown doesn't spin like a marble in its socket and make it difficult to get out, yet they aren't so long that they are difficult to remove. See Chapter 10: Common Misconceptions, for more information on wisdom teeth and how they don't cause crowding of front teeth like many people fear they do.

If your child did wear braces, this age is often a time when they stop wearing their retainers and their teeth start going crooked again. If your teeth don't naturally end up straight and perfect, but were made straight through orthodontics, then they are likely going to go crooked again if you don't continually wear a retainer. You don't have to wear a retainer all day and night, but you do have to wear it every night. If you often lose retainers or forget to put it in at night, then you can get a lingual bar. This is a metal bar that gets cemented to the back of your bottom front teeth to keep them in their current position. This tends to also keep the top front teeth in a good position as well. You never have to remember to put it in, but it can be hard to keep clean. On the other hand, a retainer is easy to keep clean, but it is hard not to lose it and remember to use.

Young Adult

As children transition from teenage years into the older years of college, they have become fairly independent. Help them regularly visit the dentist by scheduling visits for them during summer and holiday breaks. College years can be extremely busy with lots of late nights; brushing and flossing often drop by the wayside. When they are rolling into bed at 2 AM, they don't have a lot of desire to spend a couple more minutes to brush and floss. Hopefully you've helped them understand the importance of daily preventative dental care. Their habits should be strong enough to make it through their crazy years of self-discovery and growth.

Adult

By the time you reach your adult years you have pretty well cemented your oral health habits. You also are likely aware of what types of dental problems you are prone to. This is a time in your life to catch up on needed, but missed, dental treatments. You can also potentially get those aesthetic treatments you've always wanted but couldn't afford. You should proactively avoid the problems that slowly develop over time such as tooth wear.

Although tooth wear can happen for lots of reasons and occur during younger years, it often starts to show in your adult years. If severe and left unattended, it can make your smile look sixty years old when you are only forty. Tooth wear is a slow process, but like glaciers forming mountain valleys, it can make a significant change over time. Repairing this slow change can be very costly and also take multiple years to get back to normal if left for a long time. The best course is to recognize when it happens and keep the wear from progressing. Beyond this excessive wear there is also normal wear that happens to everyone, but if you avoid certain habits and excessive use of acidic foods, then you can help keep your teeth looking and feeling young for a long time. For more information on bruxism and other types of teeth wear see Chapter 6: Good Home Care to Avoid Extra Dental Visits.

There is a temporary problem that happens to many women when they get pregnant. Pregnancy significantly changes the hormones in your body. These hormones can often make the oral cavity a better place for bacteria. If you don't normally have bleeding gums and you are pregnant, suddenly your gums may start to bleed. My wife is a perfect example of this. She takes immaculate care of her teeth, but we joke that we don't need pregnancy tests. We just wait to see when her gums start bleeding and we know! Don't worry if this happens to you and you are taking good care of your mouth. As soon as your hormones return to normal, your gums will as well.

Take advantage of regular dental visits during your adult years to make sure you catch problems when they are small and to keep your gums healthy. Unhealthy gums cause bad breath and slow bone loss over time. Bone loss causes very unattractive smiles and tooth loss. Both of which are totally avoidable and very expensive to repair.

Silver Years

As a retired individual, insurance usually isn't a factor since it is often received through employers. Private insurance can be purchased, but it is almost always more cost effective to pay for things out of pocket than with insurance. Good preventative care throughout your early adult years can easily leave you with a full mouth of healthy, strong, and good-looking teeth. Gone are the days where you slowly lost your teeth until you got dentures. Not only are people losing teeth less often than they used to, but when you do lose a tooth or two, dental implants are great to restore fully functioning and aesthetically pleasing teeth.

Don't cheat yourself in your seventies with cheap fixes for dental work thinking you won't be around long enough to need a solid permanent fix. I see this too often and most people live vibrant lives long enough to have the patchwork type of dentistry come back and cost them more money in the long run and lower their quality of life. Enjoy your life! Obviously be wise with your money, but don't sacrifice your oral health. It affects so many aspects of your life, from your smile to your eating and talking. It can bother you all day every day. Instead, keep your teeth healthy, fix them as needed, and enjoy a sparkling smile that others can't help but be drawn to.

Chapter 9

Emergency Algorithm

This chapter presents an algorithm that you can use to help you decide what to do in cases of dental trauma emergencies. If you have any questions, always ask your dentist or physician. If you can't get a hold of your dentist or they do not have an emergency pager, then go to the emergency room. They can handle the immediate problems of many dental needs.

On all trauma cases:

- Handle the tooth by the crown not the root.
- Be aware that the tooth may darken due to bruising or may die and need a root canal or extraction. Some even become locked onto the bone (ankylosis).
- If your tooth doesn't return to its proper position easily, it is better to leave it alone and move the tooth later.
- You will have to monitor the tooth for ankylosis over an extended period of time.
- Often radiographs will need to be taken to evaluate what happened below the gums.

I. Tooth knocked out
   A. Primary tooth
      1. Do not replace due to high probability of ankylosis or damaging permanent tooth below it.
         a. Keep tooth and tooth fragments in skim milk or saliva of person that lost the tooth until you get to dentist.
         b. See dentist as soon as possible.
         c. The tooth will almost never be replaced due to high risk of ankylosis.
   B. Permanent tooth
      1. Replace in socket immediately if possible.
         a. After replacing, keep pressure on the bone around the tooth to help compress it back.
         b. See dentist as soon as possible.
         c. Tooth could turn dark, lose sensation, or get infected; however it often can return to be perfectly normal.
         d. If unable to replace into socket immediately, place your tooth in skim milk or saliva of person that lost the tooth. The sooner you get the tooth back in the socket, the better the outcome of the tooth will be.
II. Intrusion (tooth pushed into bone)
   A. Primary tooth
      1. Leave tooth alone.
      2. Go to dentist to have the tooth evaluated as soon as possible; it will likely be taken out.
      3. If there is no major trauma to bone, then it will likely be monitored until it comes back out to a natural position and falls out normally. It must also be monitored for possibly ankylosis or infection (abscess).
   B. Permanent tooth
      1. Leave the tooth alone.

    2. See dentist as soon as possible.

    3. It will likely be left alone to see if it comes back out on its own. If it doesn't, you may need braces to pull it back out.

III. Extrusion (tooth moved out of socket slightly, but did not come completely out)

  A. Primary

    1. See dentist as soon as possible.

    2. If slightly extruded and not very sore, you may not have to do anything after the dentist verifies what is going on. The problem may self-correct.

    3. If it doesn't self-correct, you may need to have the tooth shaved down or moved back into a normal position with braces.

  B. Permanent

    1. See dentist as soon as possible.

    2. You will likely be sent to an orthodontist for immediate braces to move the tooth back into place.

IV. Loose Tooth

  A. Primary

    1. This happens a lot due to the physically active nature of kids and the short roots of primary teeth as they get close to falling out.

    2. If tooth will fall out soon and there is no tenderness to area around tooth, it will likely be extracted.

    3. If tooth shouldn't fall out soon and wasn't loose already it may be left in, depending on several factors that the dentist will evaluate.

    4. See dentist as soon as possible.

  B. Permanent

    1. See dentist as soon as possible.

    2. You may have fractured bone or fractured tooth. It also may be as minor as the tooth just being loosened and it will go back to normal within twenty-four hours.

V. Broken Tooth
  A. Find all pieces to rule out if any were swallowed or went down your airway.
  B. See dentist as soon as possible.
  C. If you can see blood on the broken section of the tooth that is not from somewhere else, be aware that a root canal is most likely going to be done.

Follow-up care:

- You will likely need to return in one to two weeks for all trauma cases.
- Sometimes there are problems that can't be seen or evaluated at the first visit. Don't hesitate to let your dentist know if things are not getting better.
- Teeth that go through trauma often can abscess afterward. This may or may not hurt. It could just swell and often will have a pimple-like bump on the gums. Puss will sometimes come out of the bump as well. This always needs to be seen by the dentist and often requires a root canal or the tooth to be taken out.
- Traumatized teeth can ankylose to the bone. That means the bone around the tooth may fuse to the tooth. If it is a primary tooth, this can be problematic. The same is true for permanent teeth in young people. Ask your dentist to continue to monitor this for a year or so after the initial trauma.

This chapter has focused on what to do if you or someone around you experiences some trauma to their teeth. If you experience trauma around your teeth, but do not think anything is wrong with your teeth, you can choose to go to your dentist or a physician (emergency room, urgent care, etc.). Keep in mind not all dentists have a lot of trauma training. If you have pain that has come on quickly, but isn't related to trauma, see Chapter 7: Common Dental Problems and Solutions.

Chapter 10
Common Misconceptions

Like everything else in life, there are a lot of common misconceptions about dentistry. In this chapter I will go through several of them and explain the logic and science behind what really is going on. In our information age some of these misconceptions have died out due to easily accessible information, but others have become further entrenched due to propagation of false information. This propagation is often done by people who are seeking money from the sensationalism of their false information. Some false ideas are easily shown to be false. Others are much more difficult to prove false because they have several true facts, but are distorted slightly or taken too far.

Do Wisdom Teeth Cause Crowding of Front Teeth?

A common misconception that is understandable is that wisdom teeth cause crowding of your front teeth. Sometimes even dentists (hopefully naively) will say this to encourage you to remove your wisdom teeth. The misunderstanding seems likely because kids often get braces in their teens, and then in their late teens or early twenties (around the time their wisdom teeth are coming in) they notice their lower anterior teeth have become crowded. The correlation seems obvious, but as you may have heard, correlation doesn't always mean causation. This is a good example of two things happening at the same time, but one is not causing the other. It is very difficult to move teeth, which is why braces are usually worn more than a year and a half to move teeth where they should be. A lot of force is required to move each individual tooth. If teeth moved so easily that erupting wisdom teeth would crowd front teeth, then braces would be a lot quicker and easier.

A study, which has been confirmed anecdotally by thousands of orthodontists, proved that wisdom teeth do not cause this problem. They tested the crowding in teeth in people that had their wisdom teeth taken out and those that didn't. Both groups had the same amount of crowding in their lower anterior teeth. This is most likely due to two causes. First, after people get braces in their teens, they can experience continued growth in their mandible. This pushes lower teeth into upper, larger teeth, which are harder to move. In turn this crowds the lower teeth as they need to fit into their smaller, more forward jaw position. Whatever the cause, it is good to know that your wisdom teeth don't cause crowding of anterior teeth.

Is Fluoride a Poison?

Fluoride is the most discussed dental misconception with a widely varied spectrum of opinions. It is a naturally occurring element. Its use is often recommended because it makes teeth stronger. When incorporated into the enamel of teeth, the tooth is much more resistant to cavities. Yes, fluoride is also in rat poisons as you may have heard from those who are against it. So is water. Like most natural elements or chemicals (think salt), your body needs it, but too much of it can be a bad thing.

There are two main ways that fluoride can be used to help teeth. Once a child eats a fluoride pill or swallows a fluoride drop, the body will incorporate the fluoride in place of some of the calcium while the enamel is forming. This is called ingestible fluoride. The fluoride-to-calcium bond in enamel is more acid resistant than the regular calcium-to-calcium bond. Therefore, when the bacteria are producing their acid from eating the sugars in your mouth, it won't dissolve a hole as easily and create a cavity.

Because primary (baby) teeth start to form in the womb, some people have tested adding fluoride to a pregnant mother's diet without any ill effects. If that makes you uncomfortable, you can start adding it to your baby's diet whenever you do feel comfortable. See the chart in the back of the book on calcification and development timelines for more information on tooth development. This is beneficial because it is placed throughout the entire tooth and not just skimming the outside, which is referred to as topical fluoride. All of the enamel has formed in most people by age nine, at which point taking ingestible fluoride is no longer beneficial.

Soaking the outside of the tooth (topical fluoride) is the second way fluoride can help. Basically, you are just putting fluoride on the tooth in the form of a rinse or varnish. This helps to a small degree, but not nearly as much as ingesting fluoride while the tooth is forming in the jaw. Because this second method can happen throughout life, people of all ages can get fluoride treatments at the dental office. In fact, some insurance companies have found that paying for topical fluoride treatments for everyone has lowered the amount of fillings they have to pay. Thus, this preventative measure creates a win-win situation for insurance companies and their clients. They pay less for dental work when their clients need fewer fillings. You can do the same for your family by getting periodic fluoride treatments, even if your insurance isn't paying for them.

Why is water fluoridated in many cities when it only helps children and what are the negatives? The idea to fluoridate water came from how it was actually discovered to help teeth. Cities have added fluoride to the water system to help keep children from developing bad cavities and losing many teeth in their teens. Ideally, the city would use less money by providing free fluoride drops and pills for children and keep it out of the water system.

Conversely, families that are the most likely to do a poor job of cleaning their teeth are usually the ones least likely to go and take advantage of the free fluoride programs The main negative to municipal fluoride is that it also gets incorporated into bones. Stronger bones aren't necessarily better. It makes them less flexible and they tend to break easier in certain types of impacts.

Around the year 1901 in Colorado Springs, Colorado, a dentist noticed that many of his patients' teeth were a very ugly brown, but they almost never got cavities. People were obviously very happy to not get cavities, but it was emotionally hard to have dark, ugly teeth. This condition also occurred in a few other towns, but had not been reported in medical literature or researched. This dentist, the father of modern dentistry (G. V. Black), started to document and research the condition in an effort to figure out what was causing it. After many years of research, it was finally discovered that this phenomenon transpired because of naturally occurring high levels of fluoride in the water system. Fluoride is present in most well water, but not at such high levels. Over time research was done to figure out how much fluoride was needed to get the benefit of stronger teeth without causing brown stains on teeth. Today, cities fluoridate their water systems with that level. Ask your dentist if the city water is fluoridated where you live to find out if you should supplement your children.

You might hear that fluoride is terrible and a poison. People who do the research and know the most about fluoride take it themselves and give it to their children, as do most dentists that live in non-fluoridated communities. Although municipal fluoridation may not be the best solution, getting fluoride as a child is a good thing. Studies show that fluoridating a city's drinking water is associated with a 50% to 70% drop in the level of cavities. Fluoridation of drinking water is often cited as one of the greatest public-health accomplishments of the twentieth century.

Here are the common fluoride dosages for children at various ages:
- 0.25 mg drops for ages birth to 18 months
- 0.25 mg pills or drops for ages 18 months–3 years

- 0.5 mg chewable pills for ages 3–6 years
- 1.0 mg chewable pills for ages 6–9 years

Remember that maxillary second molar crowns finish forming around age eight so giving fluoride past age nine doesn't help much. Continuing fluoride use a little longer can help the upper root to incorporate fluoride as well and this can be a good idea because many adults experience some recession that exposes a couple millimeters of root surface.

Should I Avoid Getting Dental Radiographs?

I often hear people say they don't want to get radiographs taken because they want to lower their x-ray dosage. On one hand, I can understand the need to minimize radiation. On the other hand, I don't think those people understand how much x-ray radiation they get on a daily basis and where those x-rays are coming from.

The technology cartoon blog xkcd.com created an awesome chart that shows how much radiation a person gets daily and lists some examples of unexpected places that radiation might come from. I often bring this webpage up in my practice when explaining this to people (https://xkcd.com/radiation/). For example, eating a banana is 0.1 µSv and sleeping next to someone is 0.05 µSv. A set of dental radiographs is listed as 5 µSv. That means eating 50 bananas is equal to a set of dental radiographs. Note that this dental x-ray (5 µSv) is for traditional, film-based radiographs. Modern digital ones can be as low as just 1 µSv. The average person receives 10 µSv a day from naturally occurring background radiation. If you take a flight from New York to Los Angeles you get 40 µSv. Spending a few hours on the beach will also give you a large dose of radiation. I wonder if these people that decline dental radiographs are also avoiding bananas, sleeping next to their spouse, or traveling by plane?

Will I Remember What Happens to Me If I Get Nitrous During My Visit?

Nitrous Oxide gas sedation falls within the mildest category of sedation. It helps you not be as fearful as you would be without it. Patients may feel tingling or a sense of wellbeing that makes it easy for them to laugh, thus the nickname "laughing gas." However, patients definitely remain alert. Once gas administration is discontinued, the effects terminate within seconds. It is an extremely safe medicine. Dr. Niels Bjorn followed over four million cases without finding a single death! It does have a side effect of making early delivery more likely, so pregnant women should not use nitrous gas in the dental office.

Nitrous will not make you forget what happened or make you lose your ability to be aware of what is happening to you. Despite many portrayals of the gas in media as a potential way to get unknowingly molested in the dental chair, this type of sedation will not allow that to happen. There are other sedation techniques, which could make you vulnerable to such a situation, but those are referred to as conscious sedation and use medications such as Halcion.

Are Root Canals the Most Painful Procedure to Get Done?

People unnecessarily fear getting a root canal. I'm not entirely sure where this fear came from. The pain that makes you need a root canal can definitely be the worst dental pains that a person experiences. When you get a root canal done, it can be very pain free, other than the initial injection of anesthetic. Similar to when you get a filling done, the only pain should be the poke from the needle. Once that anesthetic starts to set in, there shouldn't be any pain after that.

There are cases where it can be difficult to completely get a tooth numb. If that is the case, you can take antibiotics for a couple of days before the procedure or let the infection drain and then come back later to finish it. When it comes to painful dental procedures, I hear horror stories from adults who tell of dentists forcing extractions on them when they were kids and not totally numb. Dentistry, like medicine, has become more patient friendly. If true, hopefully these stories are a thing of the past. If it has happened recently, don't ever go back to that provider, and make sure that others know of your terrible experience.

Does Bleaching Damage My Teeth?

Technically bleaching does cause damage, but it isn't something to worry about. The majority of whitening products are acidic and will dissolve some enamel molecules, most of those will be reabsorbed back into the tooth. At the microscopic level, the small amount enamel lost is insignificant. Many foods, such as soda or juice, will do the same thing.

Tetracycline stain bleach studies give a good insight into this extremely minor decalcification from teeth whitening. The antibiotic Tetracycline used to be given to kids. It worked very well, but caused brown stains on the teeth that were forming. When the adult teeth grew in a few years later, they were brown and people were unsure of the cause. The antibiotic was eventually found to be the culprit. To try and correct the dark staining, people used the strongest whitening products available, using them several hours every day for up to six months. That is an amazing amount of whitening that would turn most people's teeth so white they would look like high-powered flashlights! In these extreme cases of bleaching, no noticeable enamel changes occurred, other than whitening of course. So, feel free to whiten away to your heart's content.

There are several other misconceptions when it comes to bleaching. Companies will stretch the stories of their products' capabilities to make others think they can get those same results.

Whitening or bleaching toothpastes do help make your teeth whiter, but not in the same way as whitening gels. Teeth get dark in two ways. The first and quicker way is to pick up stain on the outside, which is what whitening toothpastes remove. They are more abrasive than regular toothpastes and polish off external stain. The second way teeth pick up stain is internally. Internal stains take longer to build up and likewise take longer to return to normal. These stains are taken care of by gels, strips, and laser whitening treatments. The degree of whitening and duration of treatment varies greatly from one product to another. In-office bleaching often works better because it has higher concentrations of whitening ingredients than those sold over the counter.

Do Silver Fillings Cause Mercury Poisoning?

Similar to the above discussion of bleaching dissolving enamel, there is a kernel of truth to silver fillings causing mercury poisoning, but it is extremely overblown. Yes, there is mercury in silver fillings, and yes, mercury is toxic. There is almost no mercury released from the fillings once in place. There have been studies done on animals, such as sheep, to see if there is mercury in their blood. These studies are skewed because sheep grind through their teeth and replace them multiple times throughout their life. Humans only replace baby teeth with adult teeth once. Since we do not grind through our teeth like sheep do, we do not ingest our fillings like sheep do. To put it in perspective, if you eat a normal amount of seafood, you are getting more naturally occurring mercury in your body than you would by having silver fillings. Mercury is present in the environment, so it is impossible to completely avoid. Minimizing our contact with mercury is the best practice for one's life. Having a few silver fillings, especially before white composites were an option, is not a situation worth losing any sleep over.

Silver fillings are more problematic because of how they cause fractures in teeth. Silver fillings expand more than the tooth does when they get hot. Silver fillings also do not stick to a tooth so they have to be placed with undercuts. That means the hole the dentist drills is bigger at the bottom than near the surface of the tooth so that the filling cannot fall out. This creates weak points in the cusps because the base is thinner than the top. If the silver filling is big enough, the weak point will eventually break from the expansion of the silver fillings heating up and cooling down. Usually the fracture propagates straight out, but at times it can angle down. When the fracture occurs, it can cause a tooth to need a root canal or extraction. The bigger the silver filling, the more surfaces it wraps around, and the longer it has been in the tooth all increase the risk of fracture.

Furthermore, dentists wouldn't be putting silver fillings in their own mouths or the mouths of their children if they were toxic. They do so knowledgeably and accept that there is a metal filling with some mercury in their mouth. The mercury isn't mixed with the other metal ingredients until right before being placed. This converts the type of mercury from one that is liquid, which can harm you, to another type that is bound up with the other metals, which isn't released into your body.

Because there are several decades of research and improvement on composite (white) fillings, there isn't a need in most cases to do silver fillings. They cost less for the dental office to place and are used in some offices for that reason, especially in offices that focus on lower-compensating insurance plans. The primary situation where it is better to use metal fillings is when a dentist can't keep a cavity preparation totally dry. In order to have the white composite fillings stick in and bond to the tooth, they have to be placed in a dry tooth. If this isn't possible, the silver filling can be a better option because they can be placed in a wet or bloody preparation without any problems.

The important thing to remember is that although you do get some mercury in your system from the placement and removal of silver fillings, the amount is negligibly small compared to amounts you get from eating seafood, something most people would encourage you to do for health reasons. The amount of mercury is a more important detail to consider. Like water, if you get too much of it, it will kill you. Just look up "hyponatremia" if you don't believe me.

If I Avoid Candy and Sugar, Will I Avoid Cavities?

This is a good question and people often think the answer is yes. Although eating simple sugars (found in candy) and then not cleaning your teeth is the easiest way to get cavities, there are many types of sugars. Complex carbohydrates, what gives you energy, are found in many other foods such as crackers, potato chips, and bread. The complex carbohydrates break down slower and are therefore more difficult for bacteria to cause cavities, but it still happens. Especially if you leave the residue on your teeth for extended periods of time. Even natural sugars found in fruits can easily cause cavities. An example would be a healthy high school girl who is trying very hard to eat healthily by snacking slowly on raisins throughout the day. This is constantly coating her teeth with natural simple sugars. The bacteria in her mouth can use these sugars to make cavities quickly.

I don't want to scare you into never eating candy or carbohydrates. Like many things in life, you just have to be responsible. Try to avoid eating or drinking things slowly when they have sugar or carbohydrates, such as sport drinks or non-diet sodas.

What Actually Is a Cavity?

Although cavities are not a misconception, they are not well understood. Like we discussed in the previous section, most people know that sugars cause cavities, but *how* do they do it? You need three things to cause a cavity: bacteria that digest sugars and produce an acid, sugars for those bacteria, and both bacteria and sugar present on teeth for a significant amount of time. There are over three hundred different types of bacteria in your mouth. Not all of them cause cavities. The two biggest culprits are Streptococcus mutans and Lactobacillus acidophilus. Most of the other bacteria are good and considered to be part of what is called the "normal flora" of your body (common groups of bacteria in all people). The bacteria Strep mutans will digest sugars for their nutrients through fermentation and produce acid as a byproduct.

This acid will dissolve the enamel of the tooth, which allows the bacteria to migrate into this newly softened portion of the tooth. As the bacteria continues to digest the sugars, the acid continues to soften the tooth and the bacteria migrate further in. Over time this creates a soft area large enough to be seen on a radiograph or for a dental explorer (the sharp instrument used by a dentist) to stick into the otherwise hard tooth. If not taken care of, the cavity will grow larger, causing the tooth to break down. Also, the bacteria will reach the hole in the middle of the tooth where the main nerve and blood vessel travel. Once there, bacteria can easily travel down that hole to the bone below the tooth and start an infection known as an abscess. In rare cases these abscesses can lead to death via Ludwig's angina, endocarditis, sepsis, or an abscess into the brain.

Chapter 11
Dental Insurance

For most people insurance is one of the most complicated aspects of dentistry. Insurance companies are not in the business of giving money away to dentists. They have lots of checks and balances in place to make sure they only pay when it is necessary. Sometimes it feels like those checks and balances are complicated on purpose to make it very difficult to get paid for even legitimate work. If you have to deal with the insurance yourself or try to verify that things were done correctly, it can be very difficult to figure out what should be covered, how much was covered, and if everything was done as it should have been done.

Most offices will accept all dental insurances, but that doesn't mean an insurance company will pay their full prices. This can be a little difficult to understand. Basically, a provider (dentist) can be in-network or out-of-network for an insurance company. In-network means the provider and the insurance company have a contract to work as partners. Out-of-network means that a dentist can treat the insurance company's patients, but they will not pay the dentist's fees if they are higher than what they want to pay. This means that you, the patient, are responsible for the difference. When you see a dentist that is in-network, the dentist agrees to lower the fees. In return these dentists will likely get more patients because subscribers to that insurance plan usually go to offices that are in-network. If a dentist does not sign a contract and agree to lower the rates to what the insurance company wants to pay, then that dentist is out-of-network. Incidentally, even if the dental office's fees are lower, you might not have to pay extra. That doesn't happen often because insurance companies pay at rates much less than the average fees.

The above situations work for most insurance plans except a type often called DMO. This is a type of plan that only allows you to go to specific providers. There is an extra deep discount for this plan, meaning the dentist is contractually obligated to charge much less than the area average. The payout is usually so low that the dental office typically rushes through patients as quickly as possible to make it profitable. This often leads to lower quality work and especially a lower quality patient experience. Keep this in mind when choosing a dental plan. Unfortunately with this type of plan, insurance companies won't pay anything to out-of-network dentists so you can only go to the providers they suggest.

Some dental offices are not in-network for any insurance companies and are called Fee for Service. This means that you will have to submit anything done to your insurance by yourself. You pay the office whatever their fee is and then hope to get as much of it paid as possible. This can be doubly difficult because dental offices do not research whether or not your procedure will be covered. If you don't find out beforehand, you could end up getting work done that your insurance won't pay for.

Typically a dental office will know common insurance plans and have a fairly accurate estimate of whether a procedure will be covered and if so at what percentage. For example, you need two fillings; a dental office normally charges $250 for a filling. To be in-network for your dental insurance, they agree to only charge $200 for that filling. Most dental insurances cover fillings at 85 percent. The treatment plan will likely say the fillings costs $250, but there is a $50 write off. The amount billed to insurance is $200, which is covered at 85 percent, so insurance will pay $170 each and you pay $30 each. On top of all that, if this is your first non-preventative (cleaning, x-rays, etc.) treatment of the year, then you will have a co-pay around $25. So, the patient portion for the first one will actually be $55, while the insurance pays $145; the second filling will cost you $30 and the insurance will pay $170.

Additionally, dental insurances are not really insurances; they are benefit plans. Insurances are safety nets that cover the costs when you can't pay. Dental insurance does the opposite. It pays from the beginning until the costs reach a certain point and then shuts off completely. The average dental insurance will pay $1,500 a year per person; it has been at that amount since the 1970s. Imagine how much more dental work you could have done during the '70s compared to now, over forty years later.

A very frustrating thing often happens to patients if they get dental work done in two different offices without notifying the second office. For example, let's say you need to have your wisdom teeth out and go to an oral surgery clinic that specializes in same-day wisdom tooth extractions. Your dentist has suggested this for the past year, so you get it done. A month later you go to your regular dentist because a tooth has been hurting. You find out you need a root canal and a crown. Because of the pain you schedule an appointment to get the work done the next day. A couple of weeks later your insurance sends you a bill for the crown because your wisdom tooth extractions and root canal used up all of your benefits. Instead of paying for half of your $1,000 crown, you now have to pay for the entire thing!

To avoid this from happening and to take full advantage of your dental insurance, you should know the following:

- Know if your dentist is in-network for your dental insurance.
- Know how much your yearly maximum is and what treatments apply (for example orthodontics is usually separate).
- Know what your co-pay is and how often you have to pay it.

- Know if your insurance covers treatment on a calendar year (January to December) or on a separate timetable to know when your coverage resets.
- Know at what percentages various treatments are covered. This can be extremely complicated so basically know at what percentage the cleanings will be covered. This includes exam, cleaning, x-rays, and possibly fluoride. Anything more will be given to you as a choice to do at a later time and you can look up specifics from there.
- Know that your dental office can request a predetermination before you do treatment. This is where the insurance company will tell you if they will cover a treatment and if so at what percentage. The negative is that you have to wait two to eight weeks for a response. I wouldn't suggest doing this for regular and less costly procedures like fillings. The dental office should be able to accurately calculate the cost. You can do this yourself as well if you get the dental codes that insurances use to describe the exact procedure.

Once you have all that information and make sure to inform the dental office of any dental treatments done elsewhere (within the current insurance coverage year), then you should be fine. Because this is so complicated, most dental offices will do their best to give you accurate estimates. Understand that they can't know if you did work elsewhere unless you tell them. Also, insurances frequently change coverages and dental offices work with many different insurances so it can be difficult to get exact pricing. Finally, a dental insurance company may always say they didn't think your treatment was necessary. So, even if they do cover that procedure, they may find a reason to deny your case.

One such frustrating example happened to my patient when insurance denied her claim citing a congenital defect. This means that she was born with a defect. In reality, as a ten-year-old her permanent canine didn't come down far enough to push the baby canine out so it was left up in the bone. Often we extract the baby tooth and have an orthodontist attach a chain to the adult tooth to easily and quickly pull it down where it belongs. She did not have this happen and eventually that baby tooth got a cavity and had heavy wear. Canines are the teeth that take the most grinding in a normal mouth. This wear, combined with the cavity caused part of the tooth to break off. Her previous filling broke a few years later due to the large size of it (composite fillings are not as strong as porcelain). At that point we did a porcelain crown so it wouldn't break again. The insurance company denied her claim stating she had a congenital defect. I appealed the decision stating that the cavity and wear happen on adult teeth and the crown was needed because of her grinding and cavity, not because it was a primary tooth. After two denied appeals, we had to give up. It was frustrating because we had no recourse other than to drop the insurance in protest, but that would hurt all of our patients on the plan.

When you have a lot of dental needs, staging treatment can be a way to take full advantage of your dental insurance. For example, if you have lots of large, old, silver amalgams that are causing significant fractures in your teeth you don't have to replace them all in one year. Start with the ones that are most likely to break and require a crown. Replace as many of them as possible without going over your yearly maximum and leave enough to cover two yearly cleanings. Then, the next year you can do the same thing. Spreading treatment out like this can help you pay as little as possible and make things easier on your pocketbook.

What do you do when you have a lot of immediate needs that can't be spread out over time? If you can't pay for it yourself or find someone to help you, then you have to do financing. Fortunately, there are a lot of good options out there. First, ask your office if they offer in-house financing. Several offices will offer an interest-free payment plan. If not, there are many companies that offer payment plans with periods of time that are interest free.

If you don't get dental insurance through your work, you might consider getting it privately. Evaluate the cost to benefit ratio during an average year. Often it seems like you pay out more than you can possibly get in return with private dental insurance. The only way to make it profitable for the provider is to have more people paying for insurance than there are people receiving benefits. If you follow the advice in this book and don't already have several dental needs, then you should be fine not getting dental insurance. Ask your dentist if they give a no-dental insurance discount.

Chapter 12
Dental Odds and Ends

The final chapter of this book will be used to put together the remaining odds and ends to help you make informed decisions about your dental health. Hopefully this book has given you a broad understanding of how best to manage your oral health as good as it can be.

Informed Consent

This is something that is fortunately happening more and more in society today, and for good reason. Many years ago the medical community was likely to do what they felt was best. Fortunately, most of the time they were right. We understand that there isn't always one perfect answer for every person in every situation. Even if there were, it is more ethically correct to allow the patient to have a say in the decision process. Yes, the medical expert is necessary to explain the pros and cons of every option and what those options are, but ultimately it should be the patient's choice. If the medical provider doesn't feel comfortable with that decision, then the patient can find another provider who is. Both parties make a decision based on a whole understanding of the situation and only do what they feel comfortable doing. Everybody isn't going to agree every time, but everybody should do what they think is right.

One important option to always remember is that you don't have to do anything. This obviously isn't a good decision if you have an infection or other similar health problem. On the other hand it can be an acceptable option in cases where you chip off a portion of porcelain fused to a metal crown in a way that it doesn't create any problems. If the chip is only in the porcelain, a food trap isn't created, and it doesn't bother you aesthetically, then leave it. Maybe polish it, but you definitely don't need a new crown. You might not always be given that option, but remember that you have it.

Similarly, ask your dentist if there are other options you could consider that they don't offer in their office. Sometimes offices may skip options that they don't offer because they could easily spend thirty minutes discussing all the options for replacing a single tooth. You could do nothing at all and leave the space in your mouth. You could do a traditional bridge. That bridge could be made of gold, gold alloys, base metal, high noble metal, partial noble metal, all-porcelain (with several all-porcelain types such as feldspathic, Zirconium, Lithium-disilicate pressed, Lithium-disilicate milled), porcelain fused to metal with all the above options of porcelains and metals mixed differently.

You could also do a Maryland bridge, implant (with all the different materials for both abutment and crown that bridge has in addition to various types of size, shape, etching to the implant), metal framework partial, acrylic solid partial, acrylic flexible partial, single tooth saddle partial, bridge with inlays in adjoining teeth rather than full crowns (plus all material options stated for traditional bridges), etc. As you can see, there are numerous options for replacing a single tooth. Dentists will give you the most commonly used options, what they feel will most likely get you the best results, and what they are comfortable doing. You will get different treatment plans from different practices because they have differing opinions. This can leave you feeling like you weren't given adequate information when in reality you were given a good range of commonly used options. This is generally considered informed consent.

Dental Vacations

Speaking of options, one option you do have is to get your dental work done in another country, which is also known as a dental vacation. While it may be tempting to get large amounts of dental work done at much lower costs, you have to consider the risks. Getting work done in another country where the dental costs are significantly lower usually means the quality controls are not the same. This refers to both quality of the work and quality of the sanitation. I've seen a few people that have done this and the work done has ranged from atrocious to acceptable. I've never seen anyone get great dental work done. This is usually because those that do great work, even in countries where the costs are significantly lower, are charging much higher prices than those around them. I'm not saying it can't be done, but it is like finding a needle in a haystack. Also, there isn't much information to help you know if you are getting high quality work in a healthy office.

Getting veneers or crowns done is not complicated for most dentists around the world. Getting veneers or crowns to be aesthetically pleasing and done in a way that will not damage other teeth or break down prematurely is not very easy. Even dentists in the United States who have to get much more education than those in some other countries don't come out of school knowing how to do that.

Becoming and Being a Dentist

So, what do you exactly have to do to become a dentist? I didn't know until after I decided to be an orthodontist. I grew up loving math, building things with my hands, and keeping to myself. Everyone said I should be an engineer, so I went to college to be a civil engineer. After a year of college and living in Argentina for a couple of years, I decided that I wanted to look into other options. College and living in Argentina had brought out the social side in me. I had braces as a teenager and liked my orthodontists, a father and son duo. It seemed like a cool job to interact with people all day and use my hands. I did not know dental school was a prerequisite before you could be an orthodontist. The more I learned about dentistry the more I began to like the idea of being a general dentist instead.

Orthodontists primarily straighten teeth all day. It sounded too routine, even if I was interacting with a wide spectrum of people. Dentists could place fillings and do surgical treatments, such as extract root tips, gum surgeries, place implants, and other bloody procedures. That sounded a lot more exciting to me! Not only could I do those surgical procedures, but I could be creative in the way I did fillings and crowns, especially the crowns that I could now make in my own office with new technology. Now that I've been in dentistry for sixteen years, I'm very glad I made this decision. I feel like I get the joy of surgery with the pleasure of getting to know people. Being a dentist is like being a friend to many great families.

To become a dentist, you typically finish a bachelor's degree and then go to an additional four years of postgraduate education. After those eight years of post-high school education, you graduate with your DDS (Doctor of Dental Surgery) or DMD (Doctor of Medical Dentistry) depending on which type of degree your school gives out. There is no difference between the two, other than which initials follow your name. The four years of dental school are sometimes combined partially with medical schools so that you take your anatomy, pathology, histology, and other classes together. Physicians get a more in-depth education in general medicine than dentists do, but we both learn much of the same information about the body.

Dental students practice developing their hand skills for drilling on teeth or bone and creating restorations. The first year is 90% didactic (book learning) and 10% hands on. The second year is about 75/25, but has the added stress of preparing for didactic boards that you take at the end of your second year. The third year is when you see patients about 75% of the time, but still spend

25% of your time in the classroom. During the fourth year you are almost entirely seeing patients in a clinic. At the end of the fourth year, there are clinical boards to prove you can do adequate dentistry in real-life situations. Also, since you have already spent so much time doing hands-on training in dental school, there is not a residency after you graduate. Many dentists choose to do a residency to become more proficient and comfortable with treatment skills before going out into the private workforce.

What Exactly Are the Different Types of Fillings?

This would be a very long discussion if were we to go through every type of restoration that is possible. To make it easier, I will stick to the main types of fillings done today. As dental science has improved over the years, the types of fillings done have also evolved. I will go over the pros and cons of each of the major ones.

Silver

The most common type of filling for several years was an amalgam filling, commonly known as a silver filling. Silver fillings are strong and help to resist cavities forming where the filling touches the tooth. They are also very cheap. Unfortunately, they aren't aesthetically pleasing because they don't look like natural teeth and can turn dark. A silver filling also expands more than the tooth does when it gets hot. Over time, especially when it is a larger filling and extends to more than one surface, large fracture lines can occur. I probably have about one person a week come to my office with an old silver filling that caused a portion of the tooth to break off. Another negative is that because they don't stick to teeth like other restorations, the filling needs to be bigger on the bottom than the top. This makes the filling too big to fall out, but it also weakens the cusps because they are more likely to fracture near the corners of the filling on the inside of the tooth. Also, there is the small negative of the presence of mercury in these fillings.

Gold

Before composites and porcelain, there were gold crowns, gold inlays, and gold onlays. These were often done as restorations when silver fillings wouldn't work. These were the "gold standard" when it came to restorative work. They had so many positives. Similar to silver fillings, they were strong, but they had to be formed outside of the mouth before being cemented. They could also be polished very smooth and shiny, resulting in a better response of the gums when the restoration went down below the gums. They didn't look like natural teeth, but they did look better than silver fillings. The gold didn't expand as much as silver fillings either, another reason they were and still are used in big restorations.

Porcelain fused to metal

Eventually porcelain started to be used because it allowed for more realistic-looking crowns. Because porcelain wasn't very strong by itself, it was often put on top of a metal base. These types of crowns are called porcelain fused to metal. They can definitely look a lot more natural than gold crowns and have many positives. Unfortunately, they aren't as strong and can fracture or chip. That breakage almost exclusively is in the porcelain, which means the tooth stays covered. Unless the porcelain breaks in a way that causes food to stick in between two teeth or allow the tooth next to it to move into a space that used to be porcelain, then the chip or fracture isn't more than an annoyance or aesthetic compromise.

Composite

Around the 1980s some offices began to use composite as an alternative to silver fillings. There were two very significant benefits. First, the fillings were white, which allowed them to look more natural than the silver fillings. Second, because they bonded to the teeth, the preparations could be much more conservative. Silver fillings needed at least 2 mm of thickness to avoid breaking. Composites could be much smaller and didn't need undercuts to stay in the tooth. Thus, dentists could place much smaller, more conservative, and more aesthetic restorations. There has been significant improvement in strength and longevity since the early days of white fillings.

Porcelain

Last, we will mention porcelain onlays, inlays and crowns. This could be a very detailed discussion as there are many different types of porcelain with different strengths and weaknesses. Suffice it to say that these, especially the more modern versions like Lithium Disilicate and Zirconia restorations, are very strong and natural looking. Dentistry truly can work aesthetic miracles with materials like these.

Botox and Dermal Fillers

Cosmetic dentistry is an area that is rapidly growing. Like many things in our modern world, many options appear each year. It is amazing and sometimes overwhelming when you look at all the options there are now. Botox and Dermal fillers are new treatment options that dental offices are starting to offer.

Botox is where someone will inject the Botulinum Toxin into your muscle. When done properly there are not any significant risks involved. It is temporary in that it lasts from three to six months. The toxin shuts down the ability of nerves to signal muscles to work. This is used to shut off the muscles of the face for two reasons. First, it makes the muscles lose their normal, slightly flexed state and relax more so that you have less wrinkles. It also inhibits those muscles from flexing when you try to use them to avoid more significant wrinkles from showing up. Second, it can work preventatively to help keep your skin from forming permanent lines that form from long-term skin wrinkling.

People usually fear getting a frozen face, meaning the person doesn't seem to have any facial expressions. This is not a legitimate concern because modern dosage techniques have really dialed in the amounts necessary to get good results. Similarly, dermal fillers can help fill in areas like deep smile lines and enhance thin lips. Adding bulk to lips is my favorite because the effects can be so immediate and amazing! Also, dermal fillers tend to last longer than Botox. See if your dentist offers these services. Few people know the facial anatomy as well as a dentist, especially ones trained in cosmetics and facial proportions. Dentists can really help you achieve beautiful results.

Sleep Dentistry

This is another area that has experienced a surge in modern dentistry. Dentists have a long tradition of making oral appliances such as bruxism devices and snore devices. A lot of research in the past couple of decades has shown how prevalent and devastating sleep apnea can be. A dental appliance can be a great solution for someone with mild to moderate sleep apnea. Basically it will hold your jaw in a forward position at night to help keep the airway from closing off. Obstructive Sleep Apnea can cause advanced aging, terrible levels of energy, and other problems. If you are not getting to stage 4 sleep, then you are not allowing your body to dump all the repair hormones into your blood. Sleep apnea keeps waking you up due to low oxygen levels and doesn't allow you to get to stage 4. You wake up feeling tired and not very well rested. It is easy to gain weight, hard to lose weight, and puts you at a significant risk for a heart attack!

Not only are dentists helping save lives, they are helping a lot of people live much fuller and more enjoyable lives. Some dental offices will do simple sleep studies to see if you have sleep apnea. They will work with your physician for a diagnosis. If you are mild to moderate, then a dental appliance can be your best option. Severe sleep apnea patients should go with a C-PAP machine. If you can't stand to use one, then you can always fall back to the dental appliance. Another important piece of information to know is that sleep apnea isn't limited to the stereotype of large, overweight men. Although they are at a higher risk of having sleep apnea, a skinny and healthy individual can also have it. For example, I am a 6'4" man that weighs 205 pounds. I work out three to five times a week, yet I have mild sleep apnea. If you suspect it, talk with your dentist or physician. It can make a significant difference in your physical and emotional wellbeing.

Chapter 13
Conclusion

Hopefully you now feel educated and armed with the information necessary to make good dental decisions for yourself and your family. Remember to use the extra documents in the appendix in addition to all the information in this book.

Good dental health is important every day of your life. Every time you smile you can smile with confidence knowing that your smile is attractive. Every time you eat, you can eat pain free. Furthermore, you won't have avoidable pains throughout the day, especially debilitating pains that stop you in your tracks.

Here's to a happy life and a happy smile!

For updates and corrections, see my website: www.insidersguidetodentistry.com.

Dr. Carson Calderwood

Appendix A
Definitions

- **Abfraction:** wear on a tooth near the gingiva, on the side of the tooth that is next to the cheeks and lips (Buccal or Facial). Usually caused from bruxism or misaligned teeth that don't send chewing forces down the long axis of the tooth.

- **Abscess:** an infection that starts in the tooth and extends into the bone past the apex of the root. Usually it will not heal itself permanently without having a root canal done.

- **Abutment:** the part of an implant restoration that goes in between the crown and the implant itself. It screws into the implant and sticks out of the gums for the crown to attach onto.

- **Amalgam:** a filling, also called a silver filling because of its silver color. Amalgam is short for amalgamation, which means a combining of several different materials. Amalgam fillings have several different metals including silver and mercury.

- **Apex:** the tip of the tooth's root.

- **Bicuspid:** a tooth with two cusps, also called a premolar.

- **Bitewing:** a type of radiograph that checks for cavities on the upper and lower teeth at the same time.

- **Bridge:** a restoration that bridges the gap between two teeth, usually has a crown on the two present teeth which are connected via a fake tooth in the middle.

- **Bruxism:** trauma to teeth caused by grinding or just clenching teeth together.

- **Buccal:** the side of the tooth that faces the gums or lips. See also "facial" for anterior teeth.

- **Calculus:** calcium buildup on teeth, commonly known as tartar.

- **Caries:** a technical term for decay in a tooth or a cavity.

- **Composite:** one of two common types of white fillings. Composites are made of a plastic-type filler (usually microscopic beads) with a resin around it that bonds to tooth and itself. The filler turns hard by shining a curing light on it. Compared to porcelain, these fillings are usually much cheaper, but not nearly as strong.

- **Coping:** a thin layer of material on a crown that attaches to the tooth. It is usually stronger than the material that goes over it.

- **Crown, restoration:** a restoration that replaces the entire outside of a tooth, also known as a cap.

- **Crown, part of tooth:** The top part of the tooth (everything that is above the root) that is covered with enamel.

- **Cusp:** the part of a tooth that sticks up and looks like the peak. Molars usually have four, premolars have two, canines have one.

- **Deciduous:** a term used to describe the primary teeth.

- **Dentin:** a substance that makes up the tooth on the inside of enamel. It has nerve fibers in it, so it can be painful if not covered by enamel.

- **Diastema:** a space between teeth. Often seen between the maxillary central incisors.

- **Distal:** opposite of mesial. Both are the sides of the tooth that touch other teeth. Distal refers to the side that is closest to the back of the mouth or farther from the midline between the left and right sides of the mouth.

- **Enamel:** a very hard substance that covers the crown portion of a tooth. It has no nerves in it.

- **Facial:** the side of the tooth that faces the gums or lips. See also "buccal" for posterior teeth.

- **Frenum:** muscle fibers that attach the cheek, lips, and or tongue to other tissue. There are two main muscle fibers— the one that connects the tongue to the floor of the mouth and the one that can go in between the maxillary central incisors causing a diastema.

- **Gingiva:** soft tissue in the mouth, commonly referred to as the gums.

- **Implant:** a titanium screw placed in the bone, which gets a crown and abutment placed on top of it.

- **Incisor:** the front eight teeth, four on top, four on bottom. They incise into food when you eat, like biting off a sandwich or piece of meat.

- **Lesion:** an injury or area of diseased tissue.

- **Mandible:** the lower jaw that holds the lower teeth.

- **Maxilla:** the upper jaw that holds the upper teeth.

- **Mesial:** opposite of distal. Both are the sides of the tooth that touch other teeth. Mesial refers to the side that is closest to the front of the mouth or midline between the left and right sides.

- **Molar:** big teeth for chewing in the back of the mouth. Adults have three in each quadrant, first molar (closest to front), second molar, and third molar (also known as the wisdom tooth).

- **Occlusal:** the chewing side of a posterior tooth. Anterior teeth have a very small occlusal, often referred to as an incisal surface, which is used for tearing or cutting into food.

- **Occlusion:** the way teeth come together when you bite down or close.

- **Onlay:** a restoration that is formed outside of the mouth and cemented or bonded into place. Usually made of porcelain, but it can be made of composite or metal.

- **Palate:** the roof of the mouth.

- **Plaque:** a soft and sticky substance made up of food debris and bacteria that accumulates on teeth.

- **Porcelain:** one of two common types of white fillings. There are several different types of porcelain, but they are all usually stronger than composite. Porcelain does not directly bond to teeth, so it needs cement to bond the restoration to the tooth.

- **Premolar:** teeth in front of the molars but behind the canines. There are two in each quadrant in the mouth.

- **Primary Teeth:** the first set of teeth that grow, which are later replaced by permanent teeth (i.e., adult teeth).

- **Prophy:** (short for prophylaxis) removing and polishing the plaque and tartar off of the teeth.

- **Pulp:** the soft tissue on the inside of a tooth. Made up of a nerve and blood vessels. Removed during root canals or pulpotomies.

- **Pulpitis:** inflammation of the dental pulp.

- **Pulpotomy:** mostly done on primary teeth, it is where the pulp is removed in the crown only and left in the roots.

- **Quadrant:** if you break up each half of the mouth into another half you have a quadrant. For example, the mandible has two quadrants, the left and right sides.

- **Restoration:** any type of filling placed in the mouth, from regular filling to a bridge or implant.

- **Root:** the bottom portion of a tooth that is normally in the bone.

- **Scaling:** cleaning tartar off teeth with instruments. This is what your hygienist is doing when she is scraping your teeth.

- **Suture:** a medical term for stitches or to place stitches.

- **Tartar:** see "Calculus."

- **TMD:** acronym for Temporomandibular Joint Dysfunction, which is problems with the temporomandibular joint.

- **TMJ:** acronym for Temporomandibular Joint. This is the joint of your jaw. It is often incorrectly used to describe TMD.

- **Torus (Tori, plural):** bone extensions. In the mandible they usually occur on the lingual side of the roots around the canine and premolars. In the maxilla, it usually occurs in the middle of the hard palate, near the back of the mouth. It is not a cancerous growth.

- **Veneer:** thin restorations to cover the front of a tooth (usually made of porcelain). It is often done as a conservative, cosmetic alternative to a crown.

- **Xerostomia:** decreased saliva production that produces a dry mouth.

Appendix B
Tables

Tooth Development

	Primary Teeth				
Maxillary (Upper Teeth)	**Central Incisor**	**Lateral Incisor**	**Canine**	**First Molar**	**Second Molar**
Initial Calcification	14 weeks	16 weeks	17 weeks	15.5 weeks	19 weeks
Crown Completed	1.5 months	2.5 months	9 months	6 months	11 months
Root Completed	1.5 years	2 years	3.25 years	2.5 years	3 years
Eruption	10 months	13 months	20 months	16 months	27 months
Mandibular (Lower Teeth)	**Central Incisor**	**Lateral Incisor**	**Canine**	**First Molar**	**Second Molar**
Initial Calcification	14 weeks	16 weeks	17 weeks	15.5 weeks	18 weeks
Crown Completed	2.5 months	3 months	9 months	5.5 months	10 months
Root Completed	1.5 years	1.5 years	3.25 years	2.5 years	3 years
Eruption	8 months	13 months	20 months	16 months	27 months

Tooth Development, continued

Permanent Teeth							
Maxillary (Upper Teeth)	**Central Incisor**	**Lateral Incisor**	**Canine**	**First Premolar**	**Second Premolar**	**First Molar**	**Second Molar**
Initial Calcification	3 months	10 months	4 months	1.5 years	2 years	at birth	2.5 years
Crown Completed	4 years	4 years	6 years	5 years	6 years	2.5 years	7 years
Root Completed	10 years	11 years	13 years	12 years	12 years	9 years	14 years
Eruption	6 years	7 years	11 years	10 years	10 years	6 years	12 years
Mandibular (Lower Teeth)	**Central Incisor**	**Lateral Incisor**	**Canine**	**First Premolar**	**Second Premolar**	**First Molar**	**Second Molar**
Initial Calcification	3 months	3 months	4 months	1.5 years	2 years	at birth	2.5 years
Crown Completed	4 years	4 years	6 years	5 years	6 years	2.5 years	7 years
Root Completed	9 years	10 years	12 years	12 years	13 years	9 years	14 years
Eruption	6 years	7 years	10 years	10 years	11 years	6 years	12 years

Tooth Development, continued

Ages at which baby (primary) teeth fall out on average					
Maxillary (Upper Teeth)	Central Incisor	Lateral Incisor	Canine	First Molar	Second Molar
Falls out on average at age	6 years	6.5 years	11 years	10 years	12 years
Mandibular (Lower Teeth)	Central Incisor	Lateral Incisor	Canine	First Molar	Second Molar
Falls out on average at age	6 years	6 years	11 years	10 years	12 years